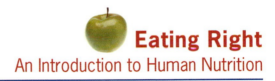

Eating Right
An Introduction to Human Nutrition

Basic Nutrition

Eating Disorders

Nutrition for Sports and Exercise

Nutrition and Weight Management

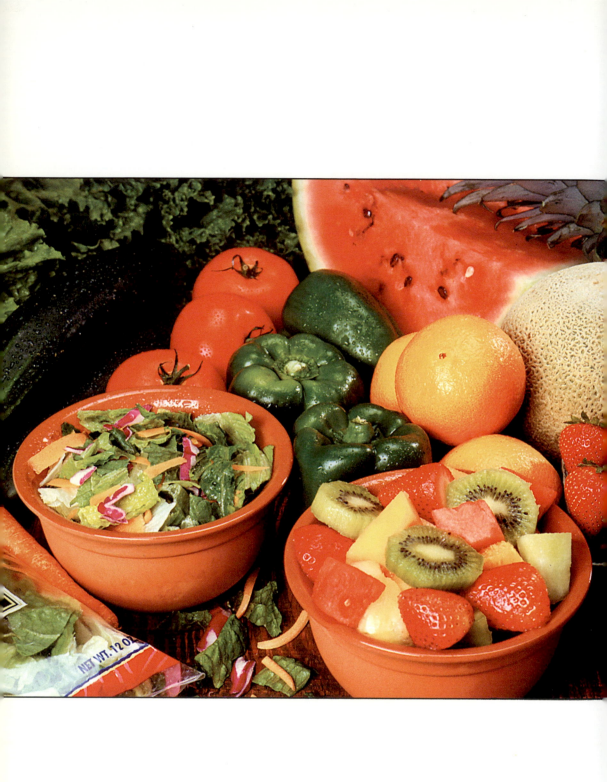

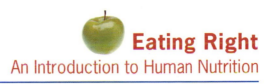

Eating Right
An Introduction to Human Nutrition

Nutrition and Weight Management

Lori A. Smolin, Ph.D.
Mary B. Grosvenor, M.S., R.D.

Preface: Lori A. Smolin, Ph.D. and
Mary B. Grosvenor, M.S., R.D.

Introduction:
Richard J. Deckelbaum, MD, CM, FRCP(C)
Robert R. Williams Professor of Nutrition
Director, Institute of Human Nutrition
College of Physicians and Surgeons
of Columbia University

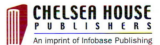

CHELSEA HOUSE
PUBLISHERS
An imprint of Infobase Publishing

Frontispiece: Maintaining weight at a healthy level is important to almost everyone. Good nutrition, including lots of fiber and fresh fruits and vegetables, is a key part of weight management.

Nutrition and Weight Management

Copyright © 2005 by Infobase Publishing

All rights reserved. No part of this book may be reproduced or utilized in any form or by any means, electronic or mechanical, including photocopying, recording, or by any information storage or retrieval systems, without permission in writing from the publisher. For information contact:

Chelsea House
An imprint of Infobase Publishing
132 West 31st Street
New York NY 10001

ISBN-10: 0-7910-7852-3
ISBN-13: 978-0-7910-7852-5

Library of Congress Cataloging-in-Publication Data
Smolin, Lori A.
    Nutrition and weight management/Lori A. Smolin and Mary B. Grosvenor.
        p. cm. (Eating right)
Includes bibliographical references.
    ISBN 0-7910-7852-3 (hardcover)
    1. Nutrition. 2. Weight loss. I. Grosvenor, Mary B. II. Title. III. Series.
RA784.S5979 2004
613.2'5dc22   2004011615

Chelsea House books are available at special discounts when purchased in bulk quantities for businesses, associations, institutions, or sales promotions. Please call our Special Sales Department in New York at (212) 967-8800 or (800) 322-8755.

You can find Chelsea House on the World Wide Web at
http://www.chelseahouse.com

Text and cover design by Terry Mallon

Printed in the United States of America

Bang 21C 10 9 8 7 6 5 4 3

This book is printed on acid-free paper.

All links and web addresses were checked and verified to be correct at the time of publication. Because of the dynamic nature of the web, some addresses and links may have changed since publication and may no longer be valid.

About the Authors

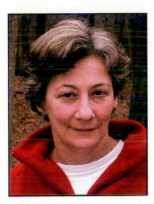

Lori A. Smolin, Ph.D. Lori Smolin received her B.S. degree from Cornell University, where she studied human nutrition and food science. She received her doctorate from the University of Wisconsin at Madison. Her doctoral research focused on B vitamins, homocysteine accumulation, and genetic defects in homocysteine metabolism. She completed postdoctoral training both at the Harbor–UCLA Medical Center, where she studied human obesity, and at the University of California at San Diego, where she studied genetic defects in amino acid metabolism. She has published in these areas in peer-reviewed journals. She and Mary Grosvenor are coauthors for two well-respected college-level nutrition textbooks and contributing authors for a middle school text. Dr. Smolin is currently at the University of Connecticut, where she teaches both in the Department of Nutritional Sciences and in the Department of Molecular and Cell Biology. Courses she has taught include introductory nutrition, lifecycle nutrition, food preparation, nutritional biochemistry, general biochemistry, and introductory biology.

Mary B. Grosvenor, M.S., R.D. Mary Grosvenor received her B.A. degree in English from Georgetown University and her M.S. in nutrition sciences from the University of California at Davis. She is a registered dietitian with experience in public health, clinical nutrition, and nutrition research. She has published in peer-reviewed journals in the areas of nutrition and cancer and methods of assessing dietary intake. She and Lori Smolin are the coauthors for two well-respected college-level nutrition textbooks and contributing authors for a middle school text. She has

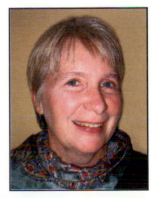

taught introductory nutrition at the community college level and currently lives with her family in a small town in Colorado. She is continuing her teaching and writing career and is still involved in nutrition research via the electronic superhighway.

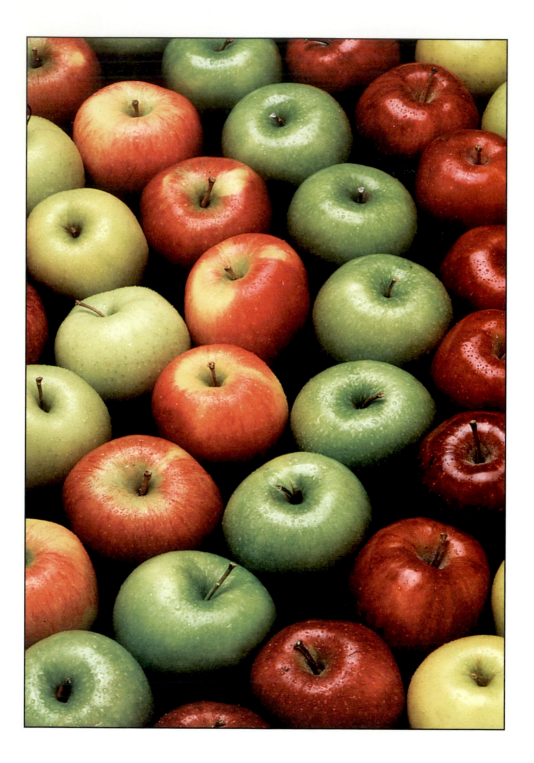

Contents Overview

Detailed Contents

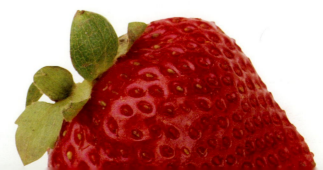

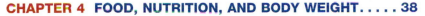

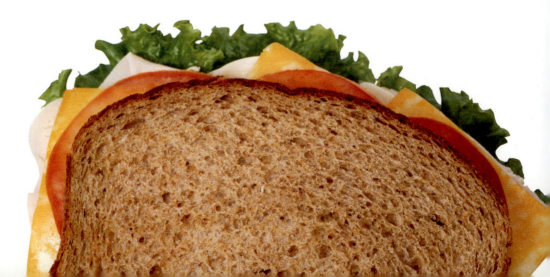

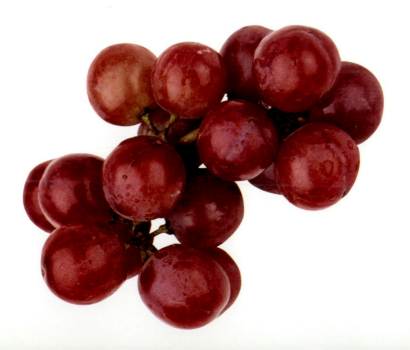

Preface

Lori A. Smolin, Ph.D.
Mary B. Grosvenor, M.S., R.D.

Fifty years ago we got our nutrition guidance from our mothers and grandmothers—eat your carrots, they are good for your eyes; don't eat too many potatoes, they'll make you fat; be sure to get plenty of roughage so your bowels move. Today, everyone has some advice—take a vitamin supplement to optimize your health; don't eat fish with cabbage because you won't be able to digest them together; you can't stay healthy on a vegetarian diet. Nutrition is one of those topics about which all people seem to think they know something or at least have an opinion. Whether it is the clerk in your local health food store recommending that you buy supplements or the woman behind you in line at the grocery store raving about the latest low-carbohydrate diet—everyone is ready to offer you nutritional advice. How do you know what to believe or, even more importantly, what to do?

Our purpose in writing these books is to help you answer these questions. As authors, we are students of nutrition. We enjoy studying and learning the hows and whys of each nutrient and other components of our diets. However, despite our enthusiasm about the science of nutrition, we recognize that not everyone loves science or shares this enthusiasm. On the other hand, everyone loves certain foods and wants to stay healthy. In response to this, we have written these books in a way that makes the science you need to understand as palatable as the foods you love. Once you understand the basics, you can apply them to your everyday choices regarding nutrition and health. We have developed one book that includes all the basic nutrition information you need to choose a healthy diet and three others that cover topics that are of special concern to many: weight management, exercise, and eating disorders.

Our goal is not to tell you to stop eating potato chips and candy bars, to give up fast food, or to always eat your vegetables. Instead, it is to provide you with the information you need to make informed choices about your diet. We hope you will recognize that potato chips and candy are not poison, but should only be eaten as occasional treats. We hope you will decide for yourself that fast food is something you can indulge in every now and then, but is not a good choice everyday. We hope you will recognize that although you should eat your vegetables, not everyone always does, so you should do your best to try new vegetables and fruits and eat them as often as possible. These books take the science of nutrition out of the classroom and allow you to apply this information to the choices you make about foods, exercise, dietary supplements, and other lifestyle decisions that are important to your health. We hope the knowledge on these pages will help you choose a healthy diet while allowing you to enjoy the diversity of flavors, textures, and tastes that food provides and the meanings that food holds in our society. When you eat a healthy diet, you will feel good in the short term and enjoy health benefits in the long term. We can't personally evaluate your each and every meal, so we hope these books give you the tools to make your own nutritious choices.

Nutrition and Weight Management discusses the current obesity crisis that is occurring in the United States. We explore the concepts of energy balance and weight control, along with genetic and environmental factors that affect these. We outline some of the health effects of being over- and underweight, and describe the pros and cons of various diets. We also provide some guidance for choosing a healthy diet.

Lori A. Smolin, Ph.D.
Mary B. Grosvenor, M.S., R.D.

Introduction

Richard J. Deckelbaum, MD, CM, FRCP(C)
Robert R. Williams Professor of Nutrition
Director, Institute of Human Nutrition
College of Physicians and Surgeons of Columbia University

Nutrition is a major factor in optimizing health and performance at every age through the life cycle. While almost everyone recognizes the devastating effects of severe undernutrition, often captured on television during famines in underdeveloped parts of the world, fewer people recognize the problem of overnutrition that leads to overweight and obesity. Even fewer are aware of the dangers of "hidden malnutrition" associated with inadequate intake of important vitamins and minerals. Unfortunately, there is also an overabundance of inaccurate and misleading nutrition advice being presented through media and books that makes it difficult for teenagers and young adults to decide for themselves what really is "optimal nutrition." This series, EATING RIGHT: AN INTRODUCTION TO HUMAN NUTRITION, provides accurate information to help people of all ages, and particularly young people, to acquire the needed tools and knowledge to integrate good nutrition as part of a healthy lifestyle. Each book in the series will be a comprehensive study in a different area of nutrition and its applications. The series will stress on many levels how healthy food choices affect the ability of people to develop, learn, and be more successful in sports, work, and in passing on good health to their families.

Beginning early in life, proper nutrition has major impacts. In childhood, good nutrition is important not only in allowing normal physical growth, but also in brain development and the ability to acquire new knowledge, both in and out of school. For example, proper dietary intake of iron is critical for preventing anemia, but just as important, it also ensures the ability to learn in the classroom and to be successful in sports or other spheres relating to physical activity. Given the major contribution of sports and exercise in improving health, it is easy to understand that nutrition truly is a partner with physical activity in promoting good health and better life outcomes.

Going into the adolescent years, many teenagers succumb to the dangers of fad diets—for example, undereating or alternatively overeating. Teens may not realize the impact of poor food choices upon their health, and, especially for girls, the risk that improper intake of vitamins and minerals will adversely impact their future families is very much underappreciated. As people mature into adults, nutritional practices have a major role in increasing or preventing the risk of major diseases such as stroke, heart attacks, and even a number of cancers. Thus, proper nutrition is an easy and cost-effective approach to achieving better growth and development, and later in markedly diminishing the chance of contracting many diseases.

Optimizing nutrition not only helps individuals but also has a major impact upon decreasing suffering and economic costs in families, communities, and nations. In the 21st century, individuals and populations will need to focus on at least three key areas. First, in promoting healthy lifestyles, nutrition needs to include a heavy concentration on diet and physical activity. Second, nutrition programs must focus on the realization that it is more important to work toward prevention rather than cure. Many of the early successes in nutrition focus on using nutrition as a treatment. We now know that improvement in nutritional status, which can easily be achieved, will have much more impact on preventing disease before it happens. Third, nutrition fits very well within the life cycle model. We know now that females who are healthy and fit *before* pregnancy are more likely to produce healthy babies and consequently healthy children. Conversely, women who have deficiencies of certain vitamins or unhealthy weights before pregnancy are more likely to have babies and children with significant health problems.

Developing countries now share the worldwide obesity epidemic. This series will help in the understanding that being overweight or obese not only changes physical appearance but also has a number of hidden dangers. For example, overweight and obesity are linked closely to rapid development of cardiovascular disease, type 2 diabetes, respiratory illnesses, and even liver disease and certain lung diseases. This "epidemic" must be fought by combined strategies using diet and physical activity. While many people today are striving to create more healthy lifestyles, they are unsure of how they should proceed. We feel that the books in this series will address these issues and provide the springboards for further thought and consideration about healthy eating.

This book in the series EATING RIGHT: AN INTRODUCTION TO HUMAN NUTRITION presents the information young people should know about nutrition, diets, and their body weight. Together with the other volumes in the series, this book targets specific areas to help the readers achieve better outcomes for themselves and their families. With the knowledge to be gained through this series, we hope that each reader will be able to enhance his/her commitment to providing a better life for himself/herself and community.

Richard J. Deckelbaum, MD, CM, FRCP(C)
Robert R. Williams Professor of Nutrition
Director, Institute of Human Nutrition
College of Physicians and Surgeons
of Columbia University

1

The Obesity Crisis

Are you worried about your weight? You are not alone. A recent survey showed that at any given time, about 45% of adult women and 25% of adult men are trying to lose weight. As large as this number seems, it is still lower than the number of people in the United States who are overweight. Currently, over 63% of adults are **overweight** and 31% of adults carry enough extra fat to be categorized as **obese**.[1] The prevalence of obesity has increased dramatically in the last 40 years; in 1960, only 13.4% of adults were obese. In just the last decade or so, the incidence of obesity has increased from 23% in 1991 to 31% today. This rise in the incidence of obesity has been referred to as an obesity epidemic. It affects both men and women and spans every age group and culture in the nation; however, there are still disparities. More women (33%) are obese than men (28%). The problem is worse among non-Hispanic black women (50%) and Mexican-American women (40%) than in non-Hispanic white women (30%). Weight problems are also increasing among children and adolescents. Ten percent of children between 2 and 5 years of age are overweight and 15% of children and teens 6 to 19 years of age are at risk for being overweight.

Why should we be concerned about the obesity epidemic? Many of us think about extra pounds in terms of how we will look in a bathing suit, but being significantly overweight is more than a matter of looks. It increases health risks and shortens life expectancy. It is estimated that 300,000 people die each year from obesity-related diseases.[2] The more overweight a person is, the greater the risk. In addition to being an individual problem, obesity is also a public health problem. It both diminishes the workforce and increases health-care costs for everyone.

WHAT IS THE CAUSE OF THE OBESITY EPIDEMIC?

Why are we getting fatter? The simple answer is that we are eating more calories than we are burning. The calories we consume in food are used to keep our bodies alive and moving. When we eat the same number of calories we use, we are in **energy balance** and

---

FACT BOX 1.1

Weight Statistics

- Adults in the Western region of the United States are less likely to be overweight.

- Married men are less likely but married women are more likely to be in the healthy weight range than single, divorced, or separated individuals.

- Women who live below the poverty level are more likely to be overweight than women in other economic groups, whereas men in this group are less likely to be overweight.

- The youngest adults (18–24) and the oldest adults (65 and over) are more likely than other age groups to be underweight.

- Being overweight is twice as common in black non-Hispanic and in Hispanic adults than it is in Asian/Pacific Islanders.

our weight stays the same. When we eat more calories than we need, our bodies store the extra, mostly as fat, and we gain weight. This ability to store extra calories as fat is beneficial when you do not know where your next meal is coming from. But it can be detrimental when food is plentiful and continuously available as it is for most of us today.

Weight Is Determined by Genes and Lifestyle

How much people weigh is determined by the **genes** they inherit from their parents and the environmental factors that affect what they eat and how active they are. A gene is a unit of information about a heritable trait that is passed from parent to child. Genetic factors explain why your body size, shape, and composition are similar to those of your parents. If one or both of your parents are obese, your risk of becoming obese is increased. However, genes do not act in isolation. They interact with environmental factors that affect lifestyle. For example, an individual with a genetic predisposition to obesity who has a limited supply of food or engages in strenuous physical labor may never become obese.

FACT BOX 1.2

Is Obesity Really an Epidemic?

The word *epidemic* is defined as a widespread outbreak of an infectious disease. Throughout human history, epidemics have devastated populations. The Black Death that first struck Europe in the 14th century killed about half the population before it ran its course. The influenza epidemic of 1918 infected a fifth of the world's population and killed between 20 and 40 million people. The virus that causes AIDS currently infects about 42 million people worldwide. Now we are faced with what has been called the "obesity epidemic." Although is is technically not an epidemic (because obesity is not an infectious disease), the increasing incidence of obesity is directly affecting a greater proportion of the population than did either the Black Death or the influenza epidemic. [a]

a Chris Forbes-Ewan. The Obesity Epidemic, Ockham's Razor National Radio. Available online at *http://www.abc.net.au/rn/science/ockham/stories/s343941.htm*.

In contrast, someone with no genetic tendency toward obesity who consumes a high-calorie diet and gets little exercise may easily become overweight.

What has changed in the United States over the last 40 years to cause this dramatic increase in the number of overweight people? The answer cannot be our genes. It takes generations for genetic changes to affect a population. The reason for our increasing girth is more likely related to changes in our environment that have led to an increase in food intake and a decrease in activity level (Figure 1.1).[3] Over the last 40 years, the availability and variety of food has increased and the need for physical activity has declined. When genetically susceptible individuals find themselves in an environment where food is appealing and plentiful and physical activity is easily avoided, obesity is a likely outcome.

Why Are We Eating More?

Americans today eat more than they did in the late 1970s.[4] Why has this occurred? A quick comparison of the food supply today with that of the late 1970s shows that the availability of tasty, high-calorie foods, the number of food choices we have, and the portions of food we eat have all increased. Today, palatable and affordable food is readily available to the majority of the population 24 hours a day in supermarkets, fast-food restaurants, and all-night convenience stores. Having more food and more food choices can lead you to eat more. Think about what makes you buy an ice cream cone. Is it because you are hungry or because the ice cream looks good? How do you know when to stop eating? Is it when your plate is empty or when your stomach is full? Your **appetite** may be triggered or inhibited by the sight, taste, and smell of food; the time of day; emotions; cultural and social conventions; and the appeal of the foods available.[5] Appetite is the reason we find room for cookies when strolling the mall or dessert after a big dinner, and it may also be the connection between an environment of plentiful food and increases in body weight.

Lifestyle changes that have occurred over the last few decades also affect how many calories Americans eat. The increasing number

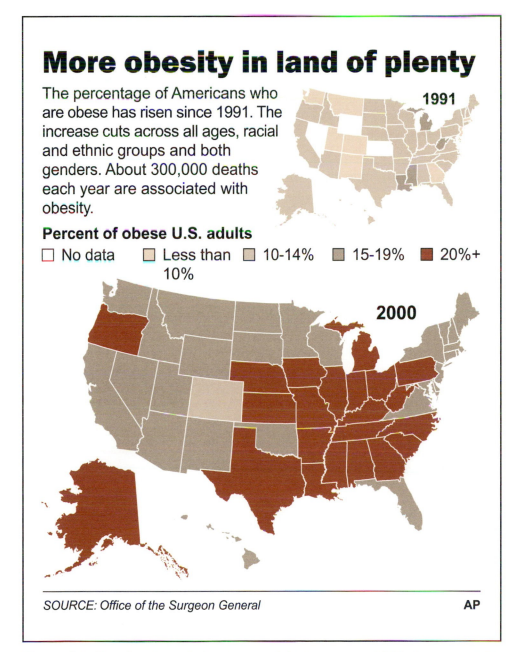

More obesity in land of plenty

The percentage of Americans who are obese has risen since 1991. The increase cuts across all ages, racial and ethnic groups and both genders. About 300,000 deaths each year are associated with obesity.

1991

Percent of obese U.S. adults

☐ No data ☐ Less than 10% ☐ 10-14% ☐ 15-19% ■ 20%+

2000

SOURCE: Office of the Surgeon General　　**AP**

Figure 1.1 More Americans today are overweight than ever. In 1991, fewer than 19% of Americans were considered obese. Just 9 years later, 22 states reported that more than 20% of their residents were obese.

of single-parent households and households with two working parents means that families have less time to prepare meals at home. As a result, prepackaged meals and fast food have become mainstays. These foods are typically higher in fat and energy than foods you would have prepared from scratch at home.

Another factor that has contributed to our increased food consumption is portion sizes. Portions have increased over time, and research has shown that providing a person with a larger serving increases the amount he or she eats.[6] Therefore, bigger portions mean we eat more. People tend to eat in units, such as one cookie, one sandwich, or one bag of chips. Increasing the size of the unit causes us to increase our intake, rather than consume only part of the unit. A look at the offerings from fast-food chains, for example, shows that portions have increased 2 to 5 times from their original size (Figure 1.2). This has been, in part, a marketing strategy. Because the cost of the food is only a small portion of what it costs a restaurant to feed you, restaurants have tried to increase sales by offering you more food for your money. Americans can't resist a bargain, so people usually spend the extra 39 cents to buy a meal that has 300 more calories. A medium order of popcorn at the movies has 16 cups

---

FACT BOX 1.3

Did McDonald's® Make You Fat?

Is the 67 grams of fat and over 1,500 calories in a burger, fries, and a shake the reason we are fat? It probably plays a part for many, but some people are going so far as to sue the restaurant industry. In July 2002, a 56-year-old maintenance worker filed a lawsuit against McDonald's®, Burger King®, Wendy's®, and Kentucky Fried Chicken®. The man claimed he had eaten fast food because it was convenient and cheap but was unaware that it could harm his health. The man weighed about 272 pounds, had survived two heart attacks, and suffered from diabetes and high blood pressure. The lawsuit argued that the companies failed to adequately inform the public of what was in their food and to provide clear warnings about the risks of a diet that includes a lot of fast food.

'Small, medium, large' now 'large, larger, largest'

A new study supports the general consensus that the size of food portions have increased in the United States. The study looked at national surveys conducted from 1977 to 1996.

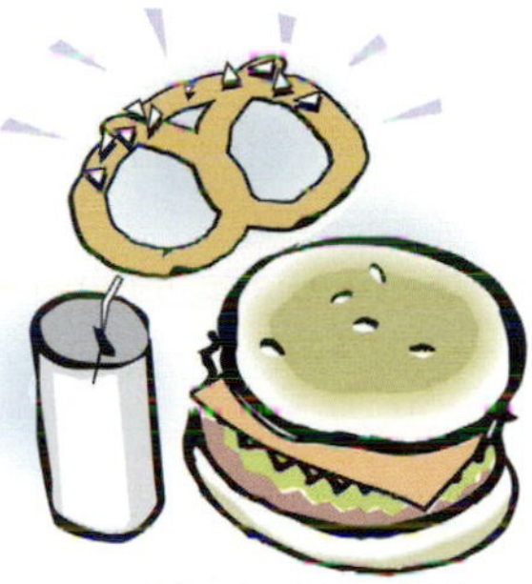

	Average portion		Percentage increase	Energy intake in kilocalories	
	1977	1996		1977	1996
Salty snacks, in ounces	1.0	1.6	60.0%	132	225
Soft drink, in fluid ounces	13.1	19.9	51.9%	144	193
Cheeseburger, in ounces	5.8	7.3	25.9%	397	533

SOURCE: Journal of the American Medical Association   AP

Figure 1.2 The more food we are served, the more we eat. Portion size has increased dramatically since the 1970s, adding to the obesity problem.

(and nearly 1,000 calories), and the drink that comes with it may add another 500 calories to your snack. A study that examined the portion sizes offered in the marketplace found that most exceed standard serving sizes set by government agencies such as the U.S. Department of Agriculture (USDA) and Food and Drug Administration (FDA) by at least a factor of 2 and sometimes as much as 8-fold.[4]

Why Are We Moving Less?

Along with changes that make it easier to eat more, there have been cultural and technological changes that have decreased the amount of energy most people use in the activities of daily American life. There are fewer adults today working in jobs that require physical labor. People drive to work in automobiles rather than walking or biking, they take elevators instead of the stairs, they use vacuum cleaners rather than brooms, and they cut the lawn with riding rather than push mowers. All of these simple changes reduce the amount of energy expended to perform the tasks of daily living. In addition, busy schedules and long days at work and commuting make people feel they have no time for active recreation. Instead, at the end of the day, Americans sit in front of televisions, electronic games, and computers—all sedentary ways to spend leisure time.

The reduction in physical activity is not restricted to adults. Many schools have reduced or even eliminated physical education programs. Social conditions that have increased crime have forced children to stay inside after school. In the 1960s, kids spent their after-school hours outdoors with bikes, balls, and friends. Today, they are more likely to spend it indoors with video games and computers. The end result is burning fewer calories than they consume and consequently gaining weight (Figure 1.3).

FACT BOX 1.4

Activity Statistics

- One in 4 adults with an advanced academic degree engages in a high level of physical activity compared to 1 in 7 of those with less than a high school diploma.

- Adults who live below the poverty level are 3 times less likely to be physically active than those in the highest income bracket.

- Married women are more likely than never-married women to engage in a high level of physical activity.

- Adults in the American South are less likely to be physically active than those in other regions.

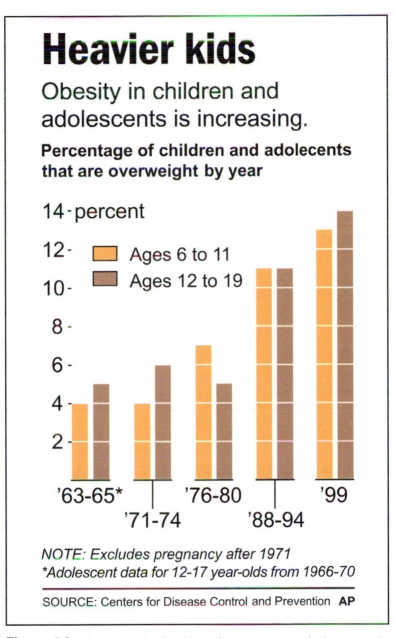

Heavier kids

Obesity in children and adolescents is increasing.

Percentage of children and adolecents that are overweight by year

14 - percent

12 - ☐ Ages 6 to 11
10 - ☐ Ages 12 to 19

'63-65*   '76-80   '99
    '71-74   '88-94

NOTE: Excludes pregnancy after 1971
*Adolescent data for 12-17 year-olds from 1966-70

SOURCE: Centers for Disease Control and Prevention **AP**

Figure 1.3 Modern technology has given us more sedentary ways to spend our leisure time, and as a result, more children are overweight and obese than ever before. More than twice as many children and adolescents were overweight in 1999 than in the 1960s.

MANAGING THE OBESITY CRISIS

Stopping the obesity epidemic involves finding a way to maintain our weight at a healthy level. For some people, this may mean avoiding weight gain as they age by making healthy food choices, controlling portion size, and maintaining an active lifestyle. For others, it may mean developing a meal and exercise plan that will allow their weight to decrease into the healthy range and stay there. For the nation as a whole, it will require the cooperation of public health programs, the medical community, and food manufacturers in order to change the environment so it is less conducive to weight gain.

U.S. Surgeon General's Call to Action

The government has addressed the rising incidence of obesity in the *U.S. Surgeon General's Call to Action to Prevent and Decrease Overweight and Obesity.*[2] This report outlines a number of strategies aimed at improving food choices and increasing physical activity. It also recognizes the importance of research that will further our understanding of the behavioral and genetic causes of obesity.

We Need to Reduce Our Portions

One of the biggest issues to address when trying to decrease intake among Americans is portion size. We have become accustomed to servings that exceed our calorie needs, and decreasing what we see as a reasonable portion will be difficult.[6] In order to accomplish this, the American public needs to be educated about appropriate portion sizes and the calorie content of different types of food. It may help to change the way portions are presented on food labels—making this information more prominent and easy to understand. Providing information about portion sizes in restaurants has also been suggested as a way to increase awareness. Food manufacturers can be involved in reeducating the public by reducing the portions they offer. Studies of the portions individuals eat have shown that we are more likely to eat the amount provided in one container than the amount listed on the label as one serving. Another way the food industry might help is to work to develop foods that have fewer calories in the same portion. For example, increasing the vegetable serving or size while reducing the fat content of a prepared meal will allow a larger serving to be consumed without increasing calories. The ultimate solution is for consumers to recognize that the value of smaller portions to their health is worth more than getting more food for less money.

We Need to Get Moving

We have become a sedentary society. We drive to work and the grocery store, take the elevator to our offices, and sit in front of computers all day. In addition, long commutes have decreased our ability to be active after work. A strategy that would help increase physical activity is to provide safe, accessible community recreational facilities for people of all ages and provide more opportunities for physical activity at the workplace.

We Need to Start Young

Currently, only about one in four teenagers nationwide takes part in some form of physical education. To increase activity level in children and adolescents, the *U.S. Surgeon General's Call to Action*

FACT BOX 1.5

Would You Pay More for Twinkies®?

One tactic that has been proposed to reduce the amount we eat of foods that are high in fat and sugar is to add a tax to junk food. Whether this would have any impact on what people eat is debatable. First of all, what is junk food? Is yogurt with 7 teaspoons of added sugar a junk food or healthy food? How about energy bars—many of which are high in sugars and fat? Even if we could define junk food, would a tax limit your intake? When you have a late night snack attack and find yourself in the 24-hour food mart in front of the donuts, Twinkies®, and HoHos®, would the price make you pass them over in favor of a piece of fruit? Probably not, although the tax might limit purchases when doing the family shopping. But, even then, would such a tax make us eat a healthier diet with more fruits, vegetables, and whole grains?

suggests that physical education be required in all school grades.[2] To improve food choices and help decrease the fat and calorie intake of school-age children and adolescents, many nutritionists have recommended that schools should reduce access to foods high in fat, calories, and added sugar by providing more healthy food options in school cafeterias and at school events. U.S. Department of Agriculture regulations prohibit serving foods of minimal nutritional value during mealtimes in school food service areas, including in vending machines, but these regulations are rarely enforced.

Small Changes Make a Big Difference

Population-based strategies to decrease food intake and increase activity levels are a good start, but they will take a long time to implement and even longer to have the effect of decreasing the number of obese people. Rather than population-wide weight loss, a more feasible goal might be to stop weight gain—halt the increase in the number of obese people that has occurred for the past few decades. Even small changes in the energy balance equation could make a big difference in arresting the increase in obesity in the population. It has been estimated that a population-wide shift in energy balance of only 100 calories a day would prevent weight gain in 90% of the population.[7] One hundred calories is the equivalent of walking for an extra 15 to 20 minutes a day (about 1 mile (1.6 km) or 2,000 steps) or reducing your ice cream serving by half a cup. Either of these or a combination is easy to do and does not require major lifestyle changes. The problem is doing it consistently from day to day. The days in which food was limited and strenuous daily physical activity was necessary for survival are not likely to return, so as a population we must learn to consciously manage our energy balance.

NOT JUST AN AMERICAN PROBLEM

Obesity is not only a problem in the United States. It is a growing concern in all industrialized countries. In England between 1980 and 1994, obesity increased from 6 to 15% in adult men and

8 to 17% in adult women. In Canada between 1978 and 1992, obesity increased from 7 to 12% in men and from 10 to 14% in women. Obesity is even becoming a problem in developing nations where we typically think of undernutrition as the main concern. In Brazil between 1976 and 1989, obesity increased from 3 to 6% in men and from 8 to 13% in women. In Thailand between 1985 and 1991, obesity rates for both men and women increased by 1%. In Western Samoa, where a strong genetic predisposition toward obesity had already made obesity rates high, it increased still further between 1978 and 1991 from 39 to 58% in men and from 60 to 77% in women.

World Health Organization Concerns

Obesity-related conditions such as cardiovascular disease, cancer, and diabetes are newly appearing, rapidly rising, or already established in every country around the world.[8] This obesity epidemic has been recognized by the World Health Organization (WHO) as one of the top ten health problems worldwide and one of the top five in developed nations. Worldwide, more than one billion adults are overweight and more than 300 million are obese.[9] Obesity levels in some developing countries are as high as those in the developed world.[8]

The causes of the growing problem of overnutrition in the developing world relate to changes that occur as economic conditions improve. With economic growth comes increased access to food and changes in diet and lifestyle patterns to ones that resemble those of developed countries. Traditional diets in developing countries are based on a limited number of foods—primarily starchy roots and high-fiber grains. As incomes increase, the diet becomes more varied and the intake of meat, fish, milk, cheese, eggs, and fresh fruits and vegetables increases.[10] Some of this change is positive. Shifts in the diet are accompanied both by increases in life expectancy and by decreases in the birthrate and in the incidence of infectious diseases and nutrient deficiencies. Along with these dietary changes come changes in lifestyle that decrease physical activity. There is a shift toward less physically demanding occupations, an increase in the use of transportation to get to work or school, more labor-saving technology in the home, and more passive leisure time. These changes in diet and lifestyle are associated with an increase in the rates of heart disease, cancer, diabetes, obesity, and childhood obesity. In countries where the economy is growing rapidly, the incidence of chronic diseases may be on the rise while infectious disease remains a common problem.[11]

International Strategies

Public health strategies to prevent and reduce obesity are necessary in both developed and developing nations around the world. The problem faced by international development agencies is more complex than it is in the United States. This is because they must promote economic growth and reduce undernutrition and infectious disease while at the same time preventing the increase in the incidence of obesity that occurs as diets become higher in fat, protein, and energy. Along with obesity, these new dietary patterns increase the incidence of chronic diseases such as heart disease, diabetes, and certain types of cancer. To address these growing health concerns, individual countries have developed public health campaigns and policies that include strategies to prevent overnutrition and promote healthy lifestyles. Nutrition goals for countries involved must emphasize the availability of a safe and adequate food supply, as well as the promotion of dietary practices to reduce chronic disease risk.

CONNECTIONS

The United States is in the midst of an obesity epidemic—more people than ever are overweight or obese. The rate of increase is particularly alarming. Body weight is determined by both genetic and environmental factors that affect food intake and activity level. The genes in a population take generations to change, so it is thought that environmental changes are the cause of the obesity epidemic. Modern lifestyles with readily available, plentiful food and the reduced need for exercise have created a situation that promotes weight gain. The Surgeon General of the United States has recommended that the American people be educated as to how to reduce their calorie intake and increase their activity level. The obesity crisis is not limited to the United States or other developed countries but is emerging in the developing world as well.

2

What Is a Healthy Body Weight?

A healthy body weight is a weight that is associated with health and longevity; a weight at which the risk of illness and death is lowest. It depends not only on how much you weigh relative to your height but also on your body composition—the proportion of weight that is lean tissue (muscles, organs, and bones) versus fat. The reason body composition is important is that the risks associated with being overweight are affected by how much body fat you have and where that fat is located on the body. Generally, we refer to the condition of carrying excess fat as being overweight; most overweight people are overfat. However, it is possible for someone to be overweight without having excess body fat. For example, a bodybuilder may weigh more than the healthy weight standard without being overfat because he or she has so much muscle. Likewise, an inactive person whose weight is in the acceptable range may have little muscle and carry an unhealthy amount body fat. In evaluating the risks associated with a given weight, it is important to assess the proportion and location of body fat.

WHAT IS YOUR BODY MASS INDEX?

Traditionally, body weight has been assessed by evaluating weight for height. Numerous tables have been developed that list healthy weight ranges for individuals of a given height and gender. The best known of these are the Metropolitan Life Insurance tables, which were developed by determining the weight at which individuals of a given sex and height live the longest (see Appendix B). However, the weights in this table may not represent the healthiest weights because they were determined when people bought insurance, not when they died. They are also based only on people who purchased life insurance, so they may underrepresent lower socioeconomic and minority groups.

The standard currently recommended to evaluate weight for height is **body mass index**, or **BMI**. BMI is determined by a mathematical equation:

$$BMI = \text{weight in kg}/(\text{height in m})^2$$

or

$$BMI = \text{weight in pounds}/(\text{height in inches})^2 \times 703$$

For example, someone who is 6 feet (1.8 meters) tall and weighs 180 pounds (81.6 kg) has a body mass index of 24.4 kg/m^2 ($180/72^2 \times 703$). A healthy body weight for adults is defined as a BMI between 18.5 and 24.9 kg/m^2. In general, people with a BMI within this range have the lowest health risks. For children and teens, who are still growing, this BMI range is not appropriate. A healthy BMI for this age group is one that falls between the 5th and 85th percentiles on the BMI-for-age growth charts (see Appendix C). **Underweight** in adults is defined as a body mass index of less than 18.5 kg/m^2, overweight is defined as 25 to 29.9 kg/m^2, and obese is 30 kg/m^2 or greater.[12] A BMI of 40 or over is classified as extreme or morbid obesity. The average BMI of adults in the United States is 26.5.[13] In people who have a BMI above 25, obesity-related diseases and increased mortality become more common (Figure 2.1).

BMI is preferred over a standard weight for height determination because it correlates better with the amount of body fat. Despite

Are you overweight or obese?

The Body Mass Index (BMI) is used to determine whether a person is at a healthy weight, overweight or obese. BMI has some limitations, in that it can overestimate body fat in people who are very muscular and it can underestimate body fat in people who have lost muscle mass, such as many elderly.

Calculating your BMI — Body Mass Index (BMI) $= \dfrac{\text{Weight (pounds)}}{\text{Height (inches)}^2} \times 703$

Body Mass Index (BMI) chart

Key   ☐ Healthy weight   ☐ Overweight   ■ Obese
         (Below 25)   (25-29)   (30+)

Weight in pounds

Height	120	130	140	150	160	170	180	190	200	210	220	230	240	250
4'6	29	31	34	36	39	41	43	46	48	51	53	56	58	60
4'8	27	29	31	34	36	38	40	43	45	47	49	52	54	56
4'10	25	27	29	31	34	36	38	40	42	44	46	48	50	52
5'0	23	25	27	29	31	33	35	37	39	41	43	45	47	49
5'2	22	24	26	27	29	31	33	35	37	38	40	42	44	46
5'4	21	22	24	26	28	29	31	33	34	36	38	40	41	43
5'6	19	21	23	24	26	27	29	31	32	34	36	37	39	40
5'8	18	20	21	23	24	26	27	29	30	32	34	35	37	38
5'10	17	19	20	22	23	24	26	27	29	30	32	33	35	36
6'0	16	18	19	20	22	23	24	26	27	28	30	31	33	34
6'2	15	17	18	19	21	22	23	24	26	27	28	30	31	32
6'4	15	16	17	18	20	21	22	23	24	26	27	28	29	30
6'6	14	15	16	17	19	20	21	22	23	24	25	27	28	29
6'8	13	14	15	17	18	19	20	21	22	23	24	25	26	28

NOTE: Chart is for adults aged 20 and older.

SOURCE: Office of the Surgeon General   **AP**

Figure 2.1 This chart is a system for determining body mass index for different heights and weights. For adults, a healthy BMI is between 18.5 and 24.9 kg/m^2. A body mass index over 30 indicates obesity. Someone with a BMI under 18.5 is underweight—which can present health problems.

this, BMI is not a perfect tool for evaluating the health risk associated with obesity. An individual with a BMI in the overweight range who consumes a healthy diet and exercises regularly may be more fit than an individual with a BMI in the healthy range who is sedentary and eats a poor diet. Or, an individual may have a high BMI but not have excess body fat. For example, someone with a large amount of muscle mass, which increases body weight, will have a high BMI, but his or her body fat and, hence, disease risk is low (Figure 2.2).

HOW MUCH BODY FAT IS HEALTHY?

What is considered a healthy body composition depends on your age and gender. At birth, the typical infant is about 12% body fat, and this percentage increases in the first year of life. During childhood, muscle mass increases and body fat decreases. During adolescence, females gain proportionately more fat and males gain more muscle mass. As adults, women continue to have more stored body fat than men. A healthy level of body fat for young adult females is between 20 and 30% of total weight; for young adult males, it is between 12 and 20%. As people age, lean body mass decreases; between the ages of 20 and 50 to 60, body fat typically doubles, even if body weight remains the same.[14] Some of this change may be prevented by physical activity.

FACT BOX 2.1

Is Your Weight in the Healthy Range?

To find out if your body weight is in the healthy range, you need to calculate your body mass index (BMI). To do this:

1) Measure your weight in pounds and your height in inches.

2) Divide your weight by your height, and then divide the answer by your height again.

3) Multiply the result by 703.

4) If you are 20 years of age or younger, use the growth chart in Appendix C to determine if your BMI is in the healthy range for someone your age.

5) If you are over 20 years of age and your result falls between 18.5 and 24.9, your BMI is in the healthy range.

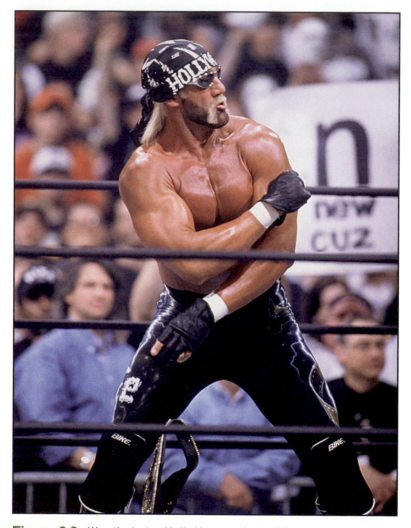

Figure 2.2 Wrestler/actor Hulk Hogan, pictured here, has a BMI that falls into the obese category, but he clearly does not carry excess body fat so his risk of disease is not increased. This is common among athletes, such as bodybuilders, since muscle weighs more than fat.

Lifestyle can affect what is considered a desirable amount of body fat. For athletes, such as distance runners, a lower percentage of body fat is desirable because this decreases the amount of weight they have to carry. Some male athletes may perform best when their body fat is only 5 to 10% and some female athletes when body fat is 15 to 20%. These athletes need enough fat to provide essential functions such as insulating the body, supplying energy reserves, and supporting normal hormonal activity, but not so much that it adds bulk. Other athletes, a professional football fullback, for instance, may need to carry extra fat to excel in his sport. Environment can also affect how much body fat is desirable. For example, people who live and work in cold climates may benefit from extra body fat to prevent heat loss.

HOW MUCH BODY FAT DO YOU HAVE?

The amount of body fat you have can be measured in a number of ways. Some of these measurements can be made in a doctor's office or at a health club; others require expensive, sophisticated equipment and are most often used in research settings.

FACT BOX 2.2

Who Stores the Most Fat?

Did you ever flop down in a chair after a big meal, thinking you felt like a beached whale? Whales are the largest mammals and have an enormous amount of body fat, but if you express their fat as a percentage of body weight, they are actually much slimmer than most humans. The largest mammal, the blue whale, weighs about 120,000 kilograms, or about 264,000 pounds. Blue whales have a layer of fat under the skin that is 6 to 8 cm thick. This represents about 15 cubic meters of fat—enough to fill your bedroom from floor to ceiling. The blue whale's percentage of body fat is only about 12% — an amount you might expect in a lean male athlete. When you feel fat, perhaps you should say you feel like a ringed seal or a lab rat! At weaning, a ringed seal pup has about 50% body fat. An adult mouse of the genetically obese Ob strain carries about 70% fat. This is much higher than the 20 to 30% body fat found in an average human. Even so, when it comes to records the humans have it. When the fattest man on record died in 1983 at age 42, he weighed 1,397 pounds (634 kg) and was estimated to be 80% body fat.

Source: The Mammal Society, Record Breaking mammals. Available online at *http://www.abdn.ac.uk/ mammal/fattest.shtml*

Skinfold Thickness

One of the easiest methods of estimating body fat is skinfold thickness. This measures the fat under the skin, or **subcutaneous fat**, which is representative of the total body fat. The measurement is done by pinching the skin and fat layer that lies over the muscles and measuring its thickness using a caliper (Figure 2.3). Skinfold thicknesses are measured at one or more locations; the most common sites for skinfold measurements are the triceps (the area over muscles on the back of the upper arm) and subscapular (just below the shoulder blade). Mathematical equations are then used to estimate body fat percentage from these measurements. The measurements can provide accurate estimates of body fat if they are performed by someone trained in the methods. However, even with a trained individual, they are difficult to perform and are less accurate for obese and elderly individuals.

Water Tanks and BOD PODs

For years, the standard for assessing body composition was underwater weighing, which involves weighing an individual both on land and under the water. The difference between a person's weight on land and his or her weight in water can be used to determine body volume and then body fat percentage can be determined using standardized equations. To measure a person's weight under water, the person sits on a scale, exhales the air from his or her lungs, and is lowered into a tank of water. Although this method is accurate, it is not practical for many people, such as small children or frail adults. A newer method for estimating body composition measures air displacement rather than water displacement to calculate body fat. The individual is placed in an air-filled chamber (known as the BOD POD) rather than in water. It is accurate and more convenient than underwater weighing.[15]

Current Flow

Your body is basically a container of salt water, so it is a good conductor of electrical current. However, body fat is a poor conductor of electricity, so it acts as a resistor to current flow. **Bioelectric Impedance Analysis** estimates body fat by measuring the rate of

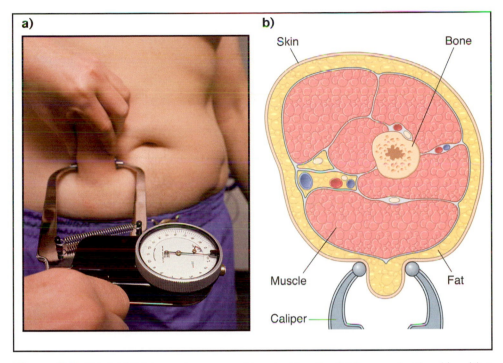

Figure 2.3 Skinfold thickness is measured by pinching the fat layer under the skin with a caliper (left). The diagram on the right shows a skinfold test done on an arm.

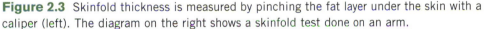

current flow through the body. This measurement is performed by directing a painless electrical current through the body with a handheld meter or a specially designed scale. Fat offers resistance and slows the current flow, so the more body fat you have, the more resistance. Bioelectric impedance techniques assume a standard amount of body water. Therefore, measurements should be done when the individual is well hydrated and the stomach and bladder are empty. Measurements are not accurate if done within 24 hours of strenuous exercise because body water has been lost in sweat.

Dilution

Body fat can also be assessed based on the principle of dilution. Because water is present primarily in lean tissue and not in fat, a detectable water-soluble substance can be ingested or injected into the bloodstream and allowed to mix with the water throughout the body. The concentration of this substance in a sample of body fluid, such as blood, can then be measured. The extent to which it has been diluted can be used to calculate the amount of lean tissue in the body, and body fat can then be calculated by subtracting lean weight from total body weight. Dilution techniques are expensive and invasive, usually requiring injections. They are used primarily for research purposes.

DEXA

A variety of sophisticated imaging techniques have been used to assess body composition. Dual-energy X-ray absorptometry (DEXA) is currently the most common. It uses low-energy X-rays to assess body composition. A single investigation can accurately determine total body mass, bone mineral mass, and body fat percentage, but it does not distinguish between visceral and subcutaneous fat. Other radiologic methods, such as CT (computerized axial tomography) scans and MRI (magnetic resonance imaging), can also be used to estimate the body fat.

ARE YOU AN APPLE OR A PEAR?

The distribution of fat in your body is important in determining the risks associated with excess body fat. Fat located around the hips and thighs is generally subcutaneous fat. Subcutaneous fat carries less risk than fat that is deposited around the organs in the abdominal region, which is called **visceral fat**. An increase in visceral fat is associated with a higher incidence of heart disease, high blood pressure, stroke, diabetes, and breast cancer. People who tend to deposit fat in their hips and thighs have been described as pear-shaped, whereas those who deposit it in their abdomens have been described as apple-shaped (Figure 2.4). Where your body fat is deposited is determined primarily by genetics, but gender, age, and lifestyle also influence where fat is stored.[16] Visceral fat storage is more common in men than women. After menopause, though, visceral fat increases in women. African-American women, who have an incidence of obesity that is 50% higher than that of Caucasian women, store

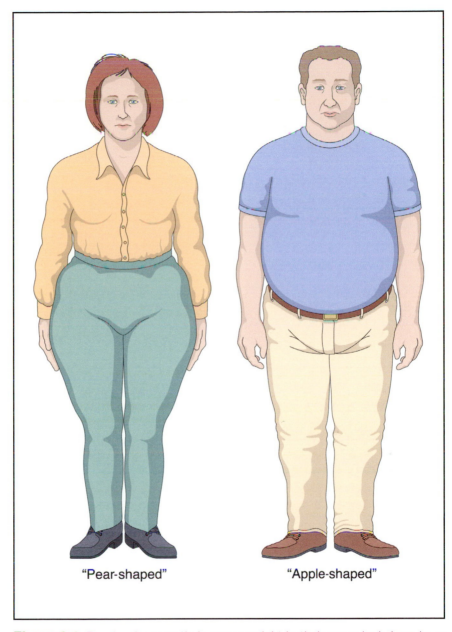

"Pear-shaped"   "Apple-shaped"

Figure 2.4 People who carry their excess weight in their upper body have been described as apple-shaped. They have a higher risk of obesity-related disease than people who carry their weight in their lower body, who have been described as pear-shaped.

Table 2.1 A High BMI and Waist Circumference Increases Disease Risk

	BMI (kg/m²)*	DISEASE RISK†	
		Men, waist < 40 inches Women, waist < 35 inches	Men, waist > 40 inches Women, waist > 35 inches
Underweight	< 18.5		
Normal weight	18.5 to 24.9		
Overweight	25.0 to 29.9	Increased	High
Obesity (class I)	30.0 to 34.9	High	Very high
Obesity (class II)	35.0 to 39.9	Very high	Very high
Extreme or morbid obesity (class III)	> 40	Extremely high	Extremely high

*   BMI = body weight (kg)/ height squared (m²)

†   Disease risk for type 2 diabetes, hypertension, and cardiovascular disease relative to individuals with a normal weight and normal waist circumference.

National Institutes of Health, National Heart, Lung, and Blood Institute. Clinical Guidelines on the Identification, Evaluation, and Treatment of Overweight and Obesity in Adults. Executive summary, June 1998. Available online at *http://www.nhlbi.nih.gov/guidelines/obesity/ob_home.htm.*

less visceral fat.[17] Stress, tobacco use, and alcohol consumption increase visceral fat deposition, whereas activity reduces it.

Distinguishing the relative amounts of visceral and subcutaneous fat requires sophisticated imaging techniques, but whether an individual carries too much visceral fat can be assessed by measuring waist circumference. In an individual with a high BMI, a greater waist circumference indicates a greater amount of visceral fat and increased health risks. For males, a BMI of 25 to 34.9 and a waist circumference greater than 40 inches is associated with increased risk. For females in this BMI range, waist circumference of greater than 35 inches increases the risks associated with being overweight (Table 2.1).

CONNECTIONS

A healthy body weight is one at which the risk of illness is the lowest. The risks associated with overweight are really due to excess body fat. The term *overweight* generally refers to excess body fat. The accepted standard for assessing body weight is body mass index (BMI). A healthy BMI for adults is between 18.5 kg/m^2 and 24.9 kg/m^2; for children and adolescents, a healthy BMI is between the 5th and 85th growth percentile for age. The proportion of body weight that is fat can be assessed by a variety of techniques, including skinfold thickness, water or air displacement, current flow, dilution, and sophisticated imaging techniques. The location of body fat can also affect the risks associated with being overweight. Subcutaneous fat, which is located under the skin, carries less risk than visceral fat, which is located around the internal organs.

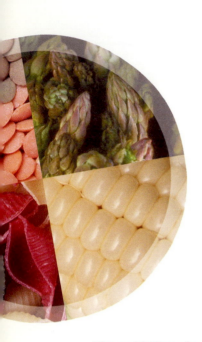

3

Body Weight and Health

The guidelines for a healthy BMI, body fat percentage, and waist circumference were developed by evaluating the body weights and compositions that are associated with the lowest incidence of disease and death. As BMI and body composition values rise above or sink below the healthy range, the risk of weight-related diseases increases. Psychological and social problems also increase with rising weight. Those who are underweight are also at risk if they do not have enough fat to provide insulation and reserves for times of illness.

BEING OVERWEIGHT INCREASES YOUR HEALTH RISKS

Carrying excess body fat increases the risk of developing chronic conditions, including high blood pressure, **atherosclerosis**, high blood cholesterol, diabetes, stroke, gallbladder disease, arthritis, sleep disorders, respiratory problems, and cancers of the breast, uterus, prostate, and colon. It also increases the incidence and severity of infectious disease and has been linked to poor wound healing and surgical complications. Being overweight increases the risks for pregnant women and their unborn children. People who gain excess weight at a young age and remain overweight throughout life have greater health risks.

Heart Disease

Obesity increases the risks of developing diseases of the heart and circulatory system. Each pound of fat adds miles of blood vessels through which the heart must circulate the blood. Extra body fat therefore increases the amount of work that the heart must perform. Extra body fat, particularly in the visceral region, also increases the risk of high blood pressure and high blood cholesterol, which contribute to the development of atherosclerosis. Weight loss can lower

---

FACT BOX 3.1

Your Heart Works Hard Enough

Your heart is a hollow, muscular organ that is about the size of a man's fist. Despite its small size, it works very hard. Every day your heart beats about 100,000 times. Each year, it beats about 35 million times, and during an average lifetime, the human heart will beat more than 2.5 billion times. The heart moves the 6 quarts (5.7 liters) or so of blood you have throughout your body three times every minute. This means that in an average lifetime, your heart pumps enough blood to fill three supertankers. But your blood doesn't go into supertankers; it travels through your blood vessels. Placed end to end, the blood vessels in your body would stretch about 60,000 miles (96,561 km), or almost three times around the Earth. If you gain weight, you grow more blood vessels to supply nutrients and oxygen to your cells. This means the heart has to work even harder to pump blood through these added miles of blood vessels. If you are 25 pounds (11 kg) overweight, you have nearly 5,000 extra miles (8,047 km) of blood vessels through which your heart must pump blood. Isn't your heart working hard enough without having to move your blood all that extra distance?

Sources: Available online at *http://www.clubs.psu.edu/FitnessPrograms/fitfacts.htm*; NOVA, Amazing Heart Facts. Available online at *http://www.pbs.org/wgbh/nova/eheart/facts.html*.

blood pressure, blood cholesterol, and the risk of heart disease. Regular exercise decreases heart disease risk by promoting a healthy body weight and composition, increasing levels of good cholesterol, and lowering blood pressure.

Diabetes

After carbohydrate-containing foods are consumed, the hormone **insulin** is secreted into the blood. Insulin allows glucose to enter cells and thus returns blood glucose levels to normal. In diabetes, either too little insulin is released or the body cells do not respond to the insulin normally. This results in the consistent elevation of blood glucose levels that is characteristic of this disease.

The incidence of diabetes in the United States is increasing along with the incidence of obesity. Most of this increase is in type 2 diabetes, the form that is caused by an insensitivity of body cells to insulin. It usually develops in adults age 40 and older and is most common in people over age 55. One reason for the increasing incidence of this disease is the advancing age of the American population. Another reason is that more Americans are overweight and sedentary. Type 2 diabetes is three times more likely to develop in an obese individual than in a non-obese individual. About 80% of people with type 2 diabetes are overweight. Type 2 diabetes is also more common in people with visceral fat, because cells in the visceral region tend to be larger and more resistant to insulin than subcutaneous fat cells.

Type 2 diabetes often occurs as part of a metabolic syndrome that includes obesity, elevated blood pressure, and high levels of blood lipids. Treatment for type 2 diabetes involves a combination of diet and exercise and sometimes medication to keep blood glucose in the normal range. Weight loss is recommended for individuals who are overweight because it improves insulin resistance and glucose tolerance.

Cancer

It is estimated that about 30% of cancers in developed countries are diet-related. Obesity increases the risk of cancers of the breast, colon, prostate, endometrium (lining of the uterus), cervix, ovary, kidney, gallbladder, liver, pancreas, rectum, and esophagus.[18] There are many ideas as to how excess body fat increases cancer risk, but the exact mechanisms are not known. Obesity is caused by complex interactions between genetics and lifestyle factors, so it is possible that some of the increase in cancer risk is due to the same factors that led to obesity and not to the obesity itself. Prudent advice is to eat a varied diet including plenty of fruits, vegetables, and whole grains; to maintain a healthy body weight with the help of regular physical activity; and to limit alcohol consumption.[19]

Gallbladder Disease

Being overweight is associated with an increase in gallstones. Gallstones are clumps of solid material that form in the gallbladder. They are typically composed mostly of cholesterol and may form as a single large stone or many small ones. These stones generally do not cause symptoms unless they become lodged in the bile ducts. This can cause pain and cramping. They can also block the passage of bile, impairing fat absorption.

The more obese a person is, the greater his or her risk of developing gallstones. Women with a BMI of 30 or higher have about twice the risk of developing gallstones as women with a BMI of less than 25. The reason that obesity increases the risk of gallstones is unclear, but researchers believe that in obese people, the liver produces too much cholesterol, which deposits in the gallbladder and forms stones. Unfortunately, gallstones are also associated with weight loss. As fat is released from body stores, cholesterol synthesis increases, making it more likely that gallstones will form.

Breathing Problems

Sleep apnea is a serious, potentially life-threatening condition characterized by brief interruptions of breathing during sleep. It occurs more frequently in people who are obese. Weight loss may decrease both the frequency and severity of sleep apnea symptoms. Asthma is also more common in obese individuals.[2]

Arthritis

Excess weight and fat can also increase the risk of developing osteo-arthritis. This is a type of arthritis that occurs when the cartilage that cushions the joints breaks down and gradually becomes rougher and thinner. As the process continues, the bones in the joint rub against each other, causing pain and reducing movement. Being overweight is the most common cause of excess pressure on the joints and it can speed the rate at which the cartilage wears down. Losing weight reduces the pressure and strain on the joints and slows the wear and tear on cartilage. Weight loss can also help reduce pain and stiffness in the affected joints, especially those in the hips, knees, back, and feet.[2]

Reproductive Concerns

Carrying excess body fat, particularly in the abdominal region, can reduce a woman's ability to conceive and to have a successful pregnancy. Weight loss, even of only 5 to 10%, can improve fertility and the outcome of future pregnancies.

Obesity is associated with irregular and infrequent menstrual cycles and decreased success with fertility treatments such as *in vitro* **fertilization**. The reasons for reduced ovulation and fertility are not completely understood, but they are believed to be caused by alterations in the metabolism and levels of estrogen and other hormones, including insulin and leptin. More estrogen is produced when there is more **adipose tissue**. In obese women, this extra estrogen may interfere with the normal cycles of estrogen released by the ovaries and hence with ovulation. Another condition that contributes to infertility in obese women is polycystic ovarian disease. This disorder is associated with being overweight, visceral fat accumulation, diabetes, and cardiovascular disease, and is characterized by a lack of ovulation or disturbed ovulation and menstrual problems.

Excess body fat can also cause problems during pregnancy. Women who begin pregnancy overweight or gain too much weight during pregnancy are at a greater risk of developing high blood pressure and diabetes during pregnancy, of having a baby with birth defects or who is **large-for-gestational-age**, and of having a miscarriage, difficult delivery, or caesarean delivery. Despite these risks, women who begin a pregnancy overweight should still gain weight during the pregnancy. Adequate weight gain during pregnancy is essential to the health of both the mother and fetus. The recommended weight gain during pregnancy is 25 to 35 pounds (11 to 15 kg) for healthy women of normal weight and about 15 to 25 pounds (7 to 11 kg) for women who are overweight at the start of pregnancy. Dieting during pregnancy is not advised, even for obese women. If possible, excess weight should be lost before the pregnancy begins or, alternatively, after the child is born and weaned. In either case, the weight loss should be gradual and accomplished by increasing activity and consuming a low-energy, nutrient-dense diet.

PSYCHOLOGICAL AND SOCIAL IMPACT OF BEING OVERWEIGHT

In addition to medical problems, psychological and social problems often occur in people who are overweight. Unlike diabetes and heart disease, obesity is a chronic health condition that is as obvious to people who see you as the clothes on your back. We live in a society that places a great deal of importance on physical appearance—and attractiveness is equated with thinness. This association makes overweight people feel unattractive. Obese individuals of every age are more likely to experience depression, a negative self-image, and feelings of inadequacy.

In American society, obesity is associated with gluttony, laziness, or both. These stereotypes are not true, but are often at the core of the prejudice and discrimination obese people may experience in the job market, at school, and in social situations. Feelings of rejection, shame, or depression are common. Overweight children are often teased and ostracized. They frequently find themselves isolated socially from their peers. Obese adolescents and adults may face discrimination in college admissions and in the work place.

Overcoming the negative self-image brought on by weight stereotypes and prejudice is made more difficult by living in a society that is sized for smaller bodies. Overweight people have difficulty finding attractive clothes and may find that airline and automobile seats are too cramped for comfort. The physical health risks of obesity may not manifest themselves as disease for years, but the emotional suffering, which is one of the most painful aspects of obesity, is felt every day.

BEING UNDERWEIGHT HAS HEALTH CONSEQUENCES

We all have body fat stores. It is essential to store some fat because it is needed for cushioning, as an insulator, and as a reserve for periods of illness. Individuals who have little stored fat have a greater risk for illness than individuals whose body fat is within the normal range. However, the health implications for someone who is naturally on the lean side are very different from the health problems seen in someone who is starving due to a food shortage or an eating disorder.

Natural Leanness

Research has suggested that being on the low side of the body weight standard may reduce your risk of diabetes, and may even increase longevity. Many lean people live to a healthy old age, but people with little energy reserves have a disadvantage when battling a medical condition such as cancer that causes wasting and malnutrition. Therefore, statistically, a low body weight is associated with an increased risk of early death.

FACT BOX 3.2

Fat Discrimination

Obese people in our society face prejudice because of their size. They may experience discrimination at work, at school, in access to public accommodations, and in getting good medical care. They are the victims of jokes; they are blamed for their condition. It is hard for them to succeed in business and in their personal lives. To try to combat this unfair treatment, groups such as the National Association to Advance Fat Acceptance have been founded. These groups work to end size discrimination, educate the public, and help overweight people to demand their civil rights.

Too little body fat causes problems at all stages of life. Low weight gains during pregnancy are correlated with an increase in low-birth-weight infants, who have a higher risk of health complications and death. For teenage girls, too little body fat can delay sexual development. In healthy but very lean female athletes, menstrual irregularities are common, causing infertility and increasing the risk of developing osteoporosis. Too little body fat in the elderly increases the risk of malnutrition. This is especially a problem when the low body weight is due to weight loss rather than a lifetime of being lean.

Starvation

In the developing world, starvation due to food shortage is a real concern. In developed countries, socioeconomic conditions may create isolated pockets of undernutrition, but severe cases of starvation are usually a result either of self-starvation due to eating disorders such as **anorexia nervosa** or of a disease such as AIDS or cancer (Figure 3.1). No matter what the cause, the effects are the same. Initially, there is a decrease in the amount of body fat, but as energy restriction continues body protein is also lost, and in children growth rate decreases. Starvation in children can lead not only to stunted growth but also to impaired mental development. As starvation progresses, its victims become weak, find it difficult to concentrate, and may have difficulty sleeping. Metabolic rate slows to decrease energy expenditure. In females, estrogen levels drop and abnormalities in the menstrual cycle occur. Substantial reductions in body weight have been shown to decrease the ability of the immune system to fight infection, increasing the risk of disease. The final stages of starvation are characterized by inactivity, apathy, and withdrawal from life. Conditions such as electrolyte imbalances, dehydration, edema, cardiac abnormalities, and infection become life-threatening.

CONNECTIONS

Carrying too much or too little body fat increases health risks. The incidence of heart disease, including hypertension, atherosclerosis, and diabetes, are increased in people who carry excess body fat.

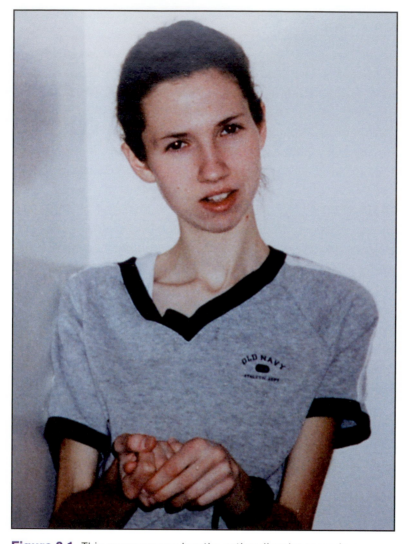

Figure 3.1 This young woman has the eating disorder anorexia nervosa, which is characterized by a restriction in food intake that leads to extreme weight loss and starvation.

Weight loss can lower blood pressure, blood cholesterol, and the risk of heart disease. The incidence of certain cancers is increased by obesity, and both obesity and weight loss increase the formation of gallstones. Breathing problems and arthritis are also more common in those who are overweight. Excess body fat affects fertility and reproductive outcome. The psychological and social problems faced by obese individuals are often more painful than the medical complications. Being too lean also carries risk. If the leanness is natural, it may have little impact, unless energy stores are needed as a reserve during illness. However, leanness due to weight loss associated with disease or a lack of food can cause serious health problems.

4

Food, Nutrition, and Body Weight

One of the first things that comes to mind when considering body weight is food. If you eat too much you will gain weight. If you eat too little you will lose weight. There are thousands of weight loss diets, programs, supplements, books, and foods on the market today that promise to help you lose weight. To understand which of these may be helpful in achieving and maintaining a healthy weight, you need to understand the basic principles of **nutrition**.

Nutrition is the study of all of the interactions that occur between people and food. It involves understanding which **nutrients** we need, where to find them in food, how our bodies use them, and the impact they have on our health. It also considers how many calories people need to keep their weight in the healthy range. An understanding of your nutritional needs can help you choose a diet with the right amount of energy and combination of nutrients to keep you healthy.

WE GET NUTRIENTS FROM FOOD

We don't eat individual nutrients, we eat foods. Food provides the body with energy and nutrients; it also contains other substances, such as **phytochemicals**, that have not been defined as nutrients but have health-promoting properties. When we choose the right amounts and combinations of food, our diet provides all of the nutrients and other substances we need to stay healthy. If we choose a poor combination of foods, we may be missing out on some **essential nutrients**. Choosing a diet that provides all of the

---

FACT BOX 4.1

What Can You Believe?

Lose 10 pounds in a week! Weight loss diets and products often make fabulous claims. Can you believe everything you read? How can you tell what is fact and what is fantasy? Generally, the rule is, if it sounds too good to be true, it probably is. The following tips offer some suggestions for figuring out whether nutritional claims are true:

- **Think about it.** Does the information presented make sense? If not, disregard it.
- **Consider the source.** Where did the information come from? If it is based on personal opinions, be aware that one person's belief does not necessarily make something true.
- **Ponder the purpose.** Is the information helping to sell a product? Is it making a magazine cover or newspaper headline more appealing? If so, the claims may be exaggerated to help the sale.
- **View it skeptically.** If a statement claims to be based on a scientific study, think about who did the study, what their credentials are, and what relationship they have to the product. Do they benefit from the sale of the product?
- **Evaluate the risks.** Be sure the expected benefit of the product is worth the risk associated with using it.

essential nutrients can be challenging because we eat for many reasons other than to obtain nutrients. We eat because we see or smell a temping food; because it's lunchtime; because we're at a party; because we are sad or happy; because it's Thanksgiving, Christmas, or Passover; and for a multitude of other reasons. In order to meet nutrient needs, we must understand what these needs are and how to choose a diet that provides them.

The Nutrients in Food

There are more than 40 nutrients that are essential to human life. We need to consume these essential nutrients in our diets because they cannot be made in our bodies or they cannot be made in large enough amounts to optimize health. Different foods contain different nutrients in varying amounts and combinations. For example, beef, chicken, and fish provide protein, vitamin B_6, and iron; bread, rice, and pasta provide carbohydrate, folic acid, and niacin; fruits and vegetables provide carbohydrate, fiber, vitamin A, and vitamin C; and vegetable oils provide fat and vitamin E. In addition to the nutrients found naturally in foods, many foods have nutrients added to them to replace losses that occur during cooking and processing or to supplement the diet. Dietary supplements are also a source of nutrients. Although most people can meet their nutrient needs without them, supplements can be useful for maintaining health and preventing deficiencies.

What Do Nutrients Do?

Nutrients provide three basic functions in the body. Some nutrients provide energy, some provide structure, and some help to regulate the processes that keep us alive. Each nutrient performs one or more of these functions, and all nutrients together are needed for growth, to maintain and repair the body, and to allow us to reproduce.

Energy

Food provides the body with the **energy** or fuel it needs to stay alive, to move, and to grow. This energy keeps your heart pumping, your lungs inhaling, and your body warm. It is also used to keep your stomach churning and your muscles working. Carbohydrates, lipids, and proteins are the only nutrients that provide energy to the body; they are referred to as the energy-yielding nutrients. The energy used by the body is measured in **Calories** or **kilocalories** (abbreviated as "kcalories" or "kcals"). When spelled with a lowercase "c", the term *calorie* is technically 1/1,000 of a kilocalorie. In some other countries, food energy is measured in joules or kilojoules (abbreviated as "kjoules" or "kJs").

Each gram of carbohydrate we eat provides the body with 4 calories. A gram of protein also provides 4 calories; a gram of fat provides 9 calories, more than twice the calories of carbohydrate or protein. For this reason, foods that are high in fat are high in calories. Alcohol can also provide energy in the diet—7 calories per gram, but it is not considered a nutrient because the body does not need it.

The more calories you use, the more calories you need to eat in order to maintain your weight. If you increase the amount of exercise you get without increasing the amount you eat, you will lose weight. Or, if you increase the amount you eat without increasing your exercise, your body will store the extra energy, mostly as body fat, and you will gain weight. When you consume the same number of calories as you use, your body weight remains the same—this is called energy balance.

Structure

Nutrients help form body structures. For example, the minerals calcium and phosphorus make our bones and teeth hard. Protein forms the structure of our muscles and lipids are the major component of our body fat. Water is a structural nutrient because it plumps up our cells, giving them shape.

Regulation

Nutrients are also important regulators of body functions. All of the processes that occur in our bodies, from the breakdown of carbohydrate and fat to provide energy, to the building of bone and muscle to form body structures, must be regulated in order to allow the body to function normally. For instance, the chemical reactions that maintain body temperature at 98.6°F (37°C) must be regulated or body temperature will rise above or fall below the healthy range. Many different nutrients are important in regulating **homeostasis** in the body. Carbohydrates help label proteins that must be removed from the blood. Water helps regulate body temperature. Lipids are needed to make regulatory molecules called **hormones**, and certain protein molecules, vitamins, and minerals help regulate the rate of chemical reactions within the body.

Getting Nutrients to Your Cells

The food we eat must be broken down and the nutrients must be transported into the body in order for them to be useful. **Digestion** breaks food into small molecules and **absorption** brings these substances into the body so they can be transported to the cells that need them.

The digestive system is responsible for the digestion and absorption of food (Figure 4.1). The main part of this system is the gastrointestinal tract, also called the GI tract. This hollow tube starts at the mouth. From there, food passes down the esophagus into the stomach and then on to the small intestine. Rhythmic contractions of the smooth muscles that line the GI tract help mix food and propel it along. Substances, such as **mucus** and **enzymes**, are secreted into the gastrointestinal tract to help with the movement and digestion of food. The digestive system also secretes hormones into the blood that help regulate GI activity. Most of the digestion and absorption of nutrients occurs in the small intestine. Absorbed nutrients are transported in the blood to the cells where they are needed. Anything that is not absorbed passes into the large intestine. Here, some nutrients can be absorbed and wastes are prepared for elimination.

How Your Body Uses Nutrients

Once inside body cells, carbohydrates, lipids, and proteins are

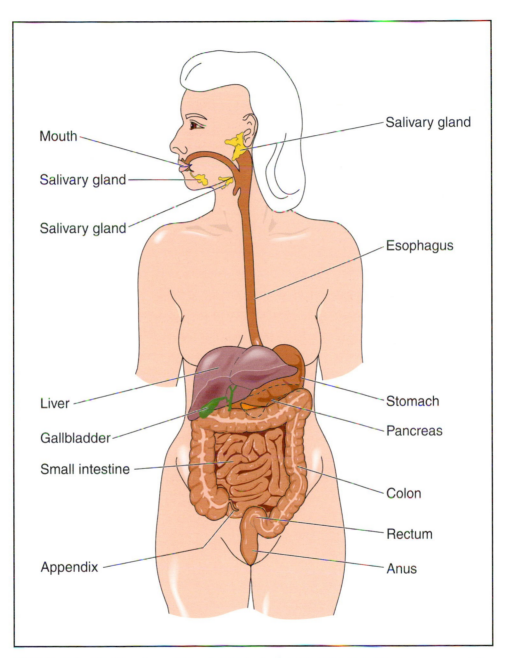

Mouth

Salivary gland

Salivary gland

Salivary gland

Esophagus

Liver

Gallbladder

Small intestine

Appendix

Stomach

Pancreas

Colon

Rectum

Anus

Figure 4.1 The digestive system is made up of the gastrointestinal (GI) tract and the accessory organs that aid digestion. The digestive system breaks food and other nutrients into pieces small enough for the body to absorb.

involved in chemical reactions that allow them to be used for energy or to build other substances that the human body needs. The sum of these chemical reactions that occur inside body cells is called **metabolism**. The chemical reactions of metabolism can synthesize

---

FACT BOX 4.2

Bacteria In Your Intestine

Did you know that your large intestine is home to several hundred species of bacteria? You provide them with a nice warm home with lots of food and they do you some favors in return—if they are the right kind. These bacteria help you digest and absorb essential nutrients; synthesize some vitamins; and process harmful substances, such as ammonia, thus reducing levels in the blood. They are important for protecting the intestines against disease, making the cells in the large intestine grow properly, and helping your body digest quickly and efficiently. A healthy population of intestinal bacteria may also help prevent constipation, flatulence, and too much acid in your stomach. However, if the wrong bacteria take over, you could get diarrhea, infections, and perhaps have an increased risk of cancer.

How can you make sure the right bacteria are growing in your gut? One way is to eat the bacteria. This is referred to as probiotic therapy. Live bacteria are found in foods such as yogurt and acidophilus milk and can be bought in tablet or liquid form. One problem with probiotic therapy is that the bacteria are washed out of the colon if you stop eating them. A second way to modify the bacteria in your gut is to eat foods or other substances that encourage the growth of particular types of bacteria. Substances that go into the large intestine without being digested and serve as food for these bacteria are called prebiotics. Prebiotics are sold as dietary supplements—but don't run to the store just yet. For most of us, eating a nutritious diet helps us maintain a healthy population of intestinal bacteria. Our understanding of how probiotics and prebiotics can be used to treat disease and promote health is still in its early stages.

the molecules needed to form body structures such as muscles, nerves, and bones. The reactions of metabolism also break down carbohydrates, lipids, and proteins to yield energy in the form of **ATP** (**adenosine triphosphate**). ATP is a molecule that is used by cells as an energy source to do work, such as to pump blood, contract muscles, or synthesize new body tissue. The production and use of ATP will be discussed more in the next chapter.

THE SIX CLASSES OF NUTRIENTS

The nutrients we need come from six different classes: carbohydrates, lipids, protein, water, vitamins, and minerals. Each class, with the exception of water, contains a variety of different molecules that the body uses in different ways. Some classes of nutrients are needed in relatively large amounts whereas others meet needs when only tiny amounts are consumed. Carbohydrates, lipids, protein, and water are often referred to as **macronutrients** because they are required in the diet in relatively large amounts. Vitamins and minerals are referred to as **micronutrients** because they are needed in just small amounts in the diet.

Carbohydrates

Carbohydrates include **sugars**, **starches**, and **fiber**. Sugars are the simplest form of carbohydrate. They taste sweet and are found in fruit, milk, and added sugars like honey and table sugar. Starches are made of multiple sugar units linked together. They do not taste sweet, and are found in cereals, grains, and starchy vegetables like potatoes. Starches and sugars are good sources of energy in the diet. Most fibers are also carbohydrates. Good sources of fiber include whole grains, legumes, fruits, and vegetables. Fiber provides little energy to the body because it cannot be digested or absorbed. It is, however, important for the health of the digestive tract.

Lipids

Lipids are commonly called fats. Fat is a concentrated source of energy in our diet and in our bodies. Most of the fat in our diet and in our bodies is in the form of **triglycerides**. Each triglyceride contains three **fatty acids**. Fatty acids are basically chains of carbon atoms. Depending on how these carbons are linked together, fats are classified as either **saturated** or **unsaturated**. Saturated fats are found mostly in animal products such as meat, milk, and butter. Unsaturated fats in our diets come from vegetable oils. Small amounts of certain unsaturated fatty acids are essential in the diet. **Cholesterol** is another type of fat found in animal foods. Diets high in saturated fat and cholesterol may increase the risk of heart disease.

Protein

Protein is needed for growth, maintenance, and repair of body structures and for the synthesis of regulatory molecules. It can also be broken down to produce energy. Protein is made of folded chains of **amino acids**. The right amounts and types of amino acids must be consumed in the diet in order to meet the body's protein needs. Animal foods such as meat, poultry, fish, eggs, and dairy products generally supply a combination of amino acids that meets human needs better than plant proteins do. A vegetarian diet containing only plant foods like grains, nuts, seeds, vegetables, and legumes, however, can also meet protein needs.

Water

Water is an essential nutrient that makes up about 60% of the adult human body. It provides no energy but is needed in the body to transport nutrients, oxygen, waste products, and other important substances. It also is needed for many chemical reactions, for body structure and protection, and to regulate body temperature. Water is found in beverages as well as solid foods.

Vitamins

Vitamins are small organic molecules needed to regulate metabolic processes. They are found in almost all the foods we eat but no one food is a good source of all of them. Some vitamins are soluble in water and others in fat, a property that affects how they are absorbed into and transported throughout the body. Vitamins do not provide energy but many are needed to regulate the chemical reactions that produce usable energy in the body. Some vitamins are **antioxidants**, which protect the body from reactive oxygen compounds like **free radicals**. Others have roles in tissue growth and development, bone health, and blood clot formation.

Minerals

Minerals are single **elements**. Some are needed in the diet in significant amounts whereas the requirements for others are extremely small. Like vitamins, minerals provide no energy but perform a number of very diverse functions. Some are needed to regulate chemical reactions, some participate in reactions that protect cells from oxidative reactions, and others have roles in bone formation and maintenance, oxygen transport, or immune function.

HOW MUCH OF EACH NUTRIENT DO YOU NEED?

To stay healthy, adequate amounts of energy and of each of the essential nutrients must be consumed in the diet. The amount of each that you need depends on your age, size, sex, genetic makeup, lifestyle, and health status. General guidelines for the amounts of nutrients needed are made by the **Dietary Reference Intakes** (**DRIs**). The DRIs were developed by teams of American and Canadian scientists who reviewed all the current research and developed recommendations for the amounts of energy, nutrients, and other substances that will best meet needs and maintain health.[20] These recommendations are general guidelines for the amounts of nutrients that should be consumed on an average daily basis in order to promote health, prevent deficiencies, and reduce the incidence of chronic disease. The exact amount of any nutrient that an individual needs depends on his or her particular circumstances.

The DRIs

The DRIs include recommendations for amounts of energy, nutrients, and other food components for different groups of people based on age, gender, and, when appropriate, pregnancy and lactation.

The recommendations for energy intakes are expressed as **Estimated Energy Requirements** (**EERs**) (see Chapter 4 and Appendix A). The recommendations for nutrient intakes include four different types of values. The **Estimated Average Requirement** (**EAR**) is the amount of a nutrient that is estimated to meet the average needs of the population. It is not used to assess individual intake but rather is designed for planning and evaluating the adequacy of the nutrient intake of population groups. The **Recommended Dietary Allowances** (**RDAs**) and **Adequate Intakes** (**AIs**) are values that are calculated to meet the needs of nearly all healthy people in each gender and life-stage group. These can be used to plan and assess individuals' diets. The fourth set of DRI values is the **Tolerable Upper Intake Levels** (**ULs**). These are the maximum levels of intake that are unlikely to pose a risk of adverse health effects. ULs can be used as a guide to limit intake and evaluate the possibility of overconsumption. When your diet provides the RDA or AI for each nutrient and does not exceed the UL for any, your risk of nutrient deficiency or toxicity is low.

What Happens if You Get Too Little or Too Much?

Consuming either too much or too little of one or more nutrients or energy can cause **malnutrition**. Typically, we think of malnutrition as a lack of energy or nutrients. This may occur due to a deficient intake, increased requirements, or an inability to absorb or use nutrients. The effects of malnutrition reflect the function of the nutrient in the body and may appear rapidly or may take months or years to appear. For example, vitamin D is needed for strong bones. A deficiency causes the leg bones of children to bow outward because they are too weak to support the body weight. Vitamin A is needed for healthy eyes and a deficiency can result in blindness. For many nutrient deficiencies, supplying the lacking nutrient can quickly reverse the symptoms.

Overnutrition, an excess of energy or nutrients, is also a form of malnutrition. An excess of energy causes obesity. It increases the risk of developing diseases such as diabetes and heart disease. Excesses of vitamins and minerals rarely occur from eating food but are seen with overuse of dietary supplements. For example, consuming too much vitamin B_6 can cause nerve damage and excess iron intake can cause liver failure.

TOOLS FOR CHOOSING A HEALTHY DIET

Knowing which nutrients your body needs to stay healthy is the first step in choosing a healthy diet, but knowing how many milligrams of niacin, micrograms of vitamin B_{12}, grams of fiber, or what percent of calories from carbohydrate doesn't help you decide what to eat for breakfast or pack for lunch. A variety of tools has been developed to help you make these kinds of choices. Three of them—food labels, the Food Guide Pyramid, and the Dietary Guidelines for Americans— are discussed below.

Understanding Food Labels

Food labels are a tool designed to help consumers make healthy food choices. They provide readily available information about the nutrient composition of individual foods and show how they fit into the recommendations for a healthy diet.

Almost all packaged foods must carry a standard nutrition label. Exceptions are raw fruits, vegetables, fish, meat, and poultry. For these foods, the nutrition information is often posted on placards in the grocery store or printed in brochures. Food labels must include both an ingredient list and a "Nutrition Facts" panel.

Ingredient List

The ingredient list includes all of the substances used when preparing a food, including food additives, colors, and flavorings. The ingredients are listed in order of their prominence by weight. A label that lists water first indicates that most of the weight of that food comes from water. You can look at the ingredient list if you are trying to avoid certain foods, such as animal products, or a food to which you have an allergy.

Nutrition Facts

The "Nutrition Facts" portion of a food label (Figure 4.2) lists the serving size of the food followed by the total calories, calories

How to Read a
Nutrition Facts Label

Macaroni & Cheese

Start Here ➡

Nutrition Facts

Serving Size 1 cup (228g)
Serving Per Container 2

Amount Per Serving

Calories 250   Calories from Fat 110

% Daily Value*

Limit these Nutrients

	%
Total Fat 12g	**18%**
Saturated Fat 3g	**15%**
Cholesterol 30mg	**10%**
Sodium 470mg	**20%**
Total Carbohydrate 31g	**10%**
Dietary Fiber 0g	**0%**
Sugars 5g	
Protein 5g	

Get Enough of these Nutrients

	%
Vitamin A	4%
Vitamin C	2%
Calcium	20%
Iron	4%

Quick Guide to % DV

5% or less is Low

20% or more is High

Footnote

* Percent Daily Values are based on a 2,000 calorie diet. Your Daily Values may be higher or lower depending on your calorie needs:

	Calories:	2,000	2,500
Total Fat	Less than	65g	80g
Sat Fat	Less than	20g	25g
Cholesterol	Less than	300mg	300mg
Sodium	Less than	2,400mg	2,400mg
Total Carbohydrate		300g	375g
Dietary Fiber		25g	30g

Figure 4.2 Standard nutrition labels like this one appear on all packaged foods. Nutrition labels help people make informed choices about what they are eating.

from fat, total fat, saturated fat, cholesterol, sodium, total carbohydrate, dietary fiber, sugars, and protein per serving of the food. The amounts of these nutrients are given by weight and as a percent of the Daily Value. **Daily Values (DV)** are standards developed for food labels. They help consumers see how a food fits into their overall diet. For example, if a food provides 10% of the Daily Value for fiber, then the food provides 10% of the daily recommendation for fiber intake in a 2,000-calorie diet. The amounts of vitamin A, vitamin C, iron, and calcium are also listed as a percent of the Daily Value.

In addition to the required nutrition information, food labels often highlight specific characteristics of a product that might be of interest to the consumer, such as advertising that a food is "low in calories" or "high in fiber." The Food and Drug Administration (FDA) has developed definitions for these nutrient content descriptors.

FACT BOX 4.3

Watch That Serving Size!

On a hot day, a bottle of iced tea or fruit juice may be just what you need to cool off. The label says that a serving has only 100 calories. Take a closer look. The serving size is 8 ounces (0.24 liters) and the bottle contains 20 ounces (0.59 liters). So your cool gulp of iced tea may be giving you 250 calories, mostly as added sugars. People tend to eat in units—one cookie, one can, one bottle. You probably won't drink half the bottle and save the rest for later. Food manufacturers are required to use standard serving sizes on the label, but they do not have to package products according to these standards. Even if the package is clearly meant to contain multiple servings, you may not always eat or drink the amount listed. For example, if you pour yourself a cup of granola for breakfast, you are probably eating about 4 servings, for a total of over 400 calories. Pasta is also a challenge because the serving size is usually given as dry pasta. What does 2 ounces (57 g) of spaghetti look like once it is cooked? It looks like about a cup (454 g), so if you pile 2 cups onto your plate, you are getting 400 rather than 200 calories with your meal.

Food labels are also permitted to include specific health claims if they are relevant to the product. These are only permitted on labels if the scientific evidence for the claim is reviewed by the FDA and found to be factual.

The Food Guide Pyramid

The Food Guide Pyramid is a visual tool for planning your diet that divides foods into 5 food groups based on their nutrient composition. Choosing the recommended number of servings from each group and following the selection tips shown in Table 4.1 will provide a diet that meets the recommendations for an adequate diet that will help promote health and prevent disease. The shape of the Pyramid helps emphasize the recommendations for the amounts of food from each of the 5 food groups (Figure 4.3). The wide base of the Pyramid is the Bread, Cereal, Rice, & Pasta Group; choosing between 6 and 11 servings of mostly whole grains forms the foundation of a healthy diet. The range of servings allows the Pyramid to be used by people with different calorie needs. For example, a 100-pound (45-kg) sedentary woman may need only 6 bread servings, whereas a 200-pound (91-kg) boxer may need 11 servings. The next level of the Pyramid includes the Vegetable Group, of which 3 to 5 servings per day are recommended, and the Fruit Group, of which 2 to 4 servings per day are recommended. Health campaigns that promote "5-a-day" are encouraging people to meet the minimum daily Food Guide Pyramid serving recommendations of 3 vegetable and 2 fruit servings. The next level, where the decreasing size of the Pyramid boxes reflects the smaller number of recommended servings, comprises the Milk, Yogurt, & Cheese Group and the Meat, Poultry, Fish, Dry Beans, Eggs, & Nuts Group. Two to 3 servings a day are recommended from each of these groups. The narrow tip of the Pyramid includes a recommendation to use Fats, Oils, & Sweets sparingly in the diet.

The variety of foods in the Food Guide Pyramid allows it to be useful as a guide for people from diverse cultures and lifestyles. For example, a Mexican American might choose tortillas as a grain,

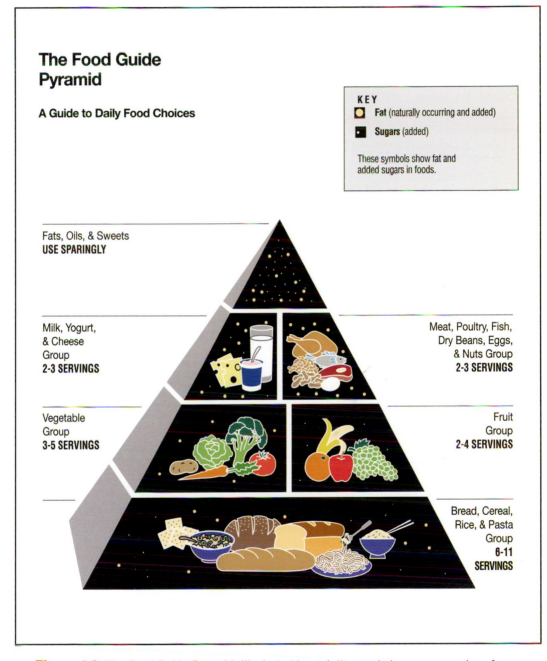

Figure 4.3 The Food Guide Pyramid, illustrated here, tells people how many servings from each food group they should include in their diets.

while a Japanese American might prefer rice; a vegetarian may choose beans from the meat and meat substitute group, while someone else might prefer beef.

Table 4.1 Servings and Selections From the Food Guide Pyramid

FOOD GROUP/SERVING SIZE	NUTRIENTS PROVIDED	SELECTION TIPS
Bread, Cereal, Rice, & Pasta (6 to 11 servings) 1/2 cup cooked cereal, rice, or pasta 1 ounce dry cereal 1 slice bread 1 tortilla 2 cookies 1/2 medium donut	B vitamins Fiber Iron Magnesium Zinc Complex carbohydrates	• Choose whole-grain breads, cereals, and grains such as whole wheat or rye, oatmeal, and brown rice. • Consume high-fat, high-sugar baked goods such as cakes, cookies, and pastries in moderation. • Limit fats and sugars added as spreads, sauces, or toppings.
Vegetable (3 to 5 servings) 1/2 cup cooked or raw chopped vegetables 1 cup raw leafy vegetables 3/4 cup vegetable juice 10 french fries	Vitamin A Vitamin C Folate Magnesium Iron Fiber	• Eat a variety of vegetables, including dark-green leafy vegetables like spinach and broccoli, deep-yellow vegetables like carrots and sweet potatoes, starchy vegetables such as potatoes and corn, and other vegetables such as green beans and tomatoes. • Cook by steaming or baking. • Avoid frying, and limit high-fat spreads or dressings.
Fruit (2 to 4 servings) 1 medium apple, banana, or orange 1/2 cup chopped, cooked, or canned fruit 3/4 cup fruit juice 1/4 cup dried fruit	Vitamin A Vitamin C Potassium Fiber	• Choose fresh fruit, frozen fruit without sugar, dried fruit, or fruit canned in water or juice. • If canned in heavy syrup, rinse fruit with water before eating. • Eat whole fruits more often than juices; they are higher in fiber. • Regularly eat citrus fruits, melons, or berries rich in vitamin C. • Only 100% fruit juice should be counted as fruit.

The Dietary Guidelines

The Dietary Guidelines for Americans is another useful tool that can help you choose a healthy diet. It is a set of recommendations on diet

FOOD GROUP/SERVING SIZE	NUTRIENTS PROVIDED	SELECTION TIPS
Milk, Yogurt, & Cheese (2 to 3 servings) 1 cup milk or yogurt 1-1/2 ounces natural cheese 2 ounces processed cheese 2 cups cottage cheese 1-1/2 cups ice cream 1 cup frozen yogurt	Protein Calcium Riboflavin Vitamin D	• Use low-fat or skim milk for healthy people over 2 years of age. • Choose low-fat and nonfat yogurt, "part skim" and low-fat cheeses, and lower-fat frozen desserts like ice milk and frozen yogurt. • Limit high-fat cheeses and ice cream.
Meat, Poultry, Fish, Dry Beans, Eggs, & Nuts (2 to 3 servings) 2–3 ounces cooked lean meat, fish, or poultry 2–3 eggs 4–6 tablespoons peanut butter 1 to 1-1/2 cups cooked dry beans 2/3 to 1 cup nuts	Protein Niacin Vitamin B_6 Vitamin B_{12} Other B vitamins Iron Zinc	• Select lean meat, poultry without skin, and dry beans often. • Trim fat, and cook by broiling, roasting, grilling, or boiling rather than frying. • Limit egg yolks, which are high in cholesterol, and nuts and seeds, which are high in fat. • Be aware of serving size; 3 ounces of meat is the size of an average hamburger.
Fats, Oils, & Sweets (use sparingly) Butter Mayonnaise Salad dressing Cream cheese Sour cream Jam Jelly	Fat-soluble vitamins	• These are high in energy and low in micronutrients. • Substitute low-fat dressings and spreads.

Human Nutrition Information Service. *The Food Guide Pyramid.* Home and Garden Bulletin No. 252. Hyattsville, MD: U.S. Department of Agriculture, 1992, 1996, revised.

and lifestyle designed to promote health, support active lives, and reduce chronic disease risks. It is organized into three tiers: the ABCs for Good Health (Figure 4.4).

The first tier, called "Aim for Fitness," includes two guidelines that recommend that we "Aim for a healthy weight" and "Be physically active each day." These guidelines are backed up by specific recommendations for body weight and activity levels.

The "Build a Healthy Base" tier offers four guidelines on choosing a variety of foods and handling these foods safely. It recommends that we let the Pyramid guide our food choices; eat a variety of grains, especially whole grains, daily; eat a variety of fruits and vegetables daily; and "Keep food safe to eat."

The last tier, "Choose Sensibly," recommends limiting intakes of certain dietary components. The first guideline—"Choose a diet that is low in saturated fat and cholesterol and moderate in total fat"—reflects the understanding that diets low in saturated fat and cholesterol may reduce the risk of heart disease. The guideline to "Choose beverages and foods to moderate your intake of sugars" is based on the fact that the consumption of sugars in the United States has been on the rise and may be affecting the incidence of chronic disease. "Choose and prepare foods with less salt" is based on research that indicates that a diet high in salt increases blood pressure in some individuals. The final guideline emphasizes the dangers of excess alcohol consumption.

CONNECTIONS

We don't eat individual nutrients; we eat food. Food provides our bodies with energy in the form of calories and nutrients, which are substances required in the diet for growth, reproduction, and maintenance of the body. The right number of calories is needed to keep weight in the healthy range and the right combination of nutrients is needed to maintain health. There are six classes of nutrients. Carbohydrates include sugars, starches, and fibers. Sugars and starches provide energy, 4 calories per gram. Fibers provide little energy because they cannot be digested by human enzymes and therefore cannot be absorbed. Lipids are a concentrated source of

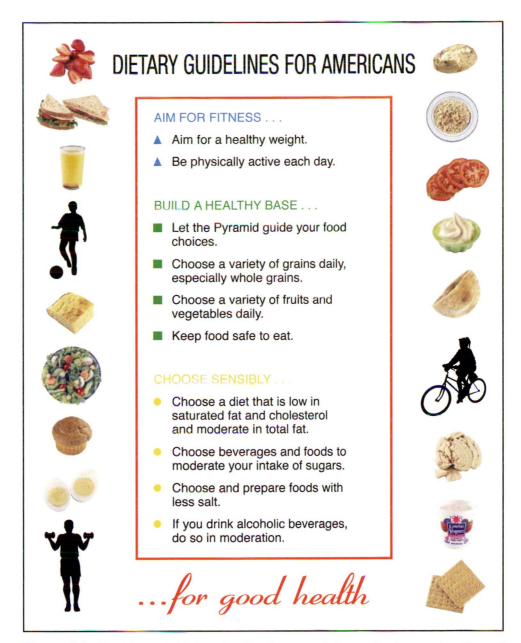

DIETARY GUIDELINES FOR AMERICANS

AIM FOR FITNESS . . .

▲ Aim for a healthy weight.

▲ Be physically active each day.

BUILD A HEALTHY BASE . . .

■ Let the Pyramid guide your food choices.

■ Choose a variety of grains daily, especially whole grains.

■ Choose a variety of fruits and vegetables daily.

■ Keep food safe to eat.

CHOOSE SENSIBLY . . .

● Choose a diet that is low in saturated fat and cholesterol and moderate in total fat.

● Choose beverages and foods to moderate your intake of sugars.

● Choose and prepare foods with less salt.

● If you drink alcoholic beverages, do so in moderation.

...for good health

Figure 4.4 The Dietary Guidelines for Americans can help people choose a healthy and sensible diet. These guidelines suggest that people get enough exercise; choose a variety of different, healthy foods; and limit their intake of certain food components, such as salt, sugar, and cholesterol.

calories in the diet and in the body, providing 9 calories per gram. They are also needed to synthesize molecules that provide structure and help regulate body processes. Proteins are made from amino acids. In the body, proteins can provide energy but are more important for their structural and regulatory roles. Water is the most abundant

---

FACT BOX 4.4

How Healthy Is the American Diet?

A healthy diet should be based on whole grains, vegetables, and fruits, with smaller amounts of dairy products and high-protein foods and limited amounts of fats and sweets. In general, the American diet doesn't meet these recommendations. The Dietary Guidelines and the Food Guide Pyramid say we should choose whole rather than refined grains, but the average American eats only one serving of whole grains per day. The Food Guide Pyramid recommends 2–4 servings of fruit, but most people eat only 1-2/3 servings each day and 48% of Americans don't consume even one piece of fruit daily. We also fall short of the 2–3 servings of dairy products recommended. Americans on average eat only 1-1/2 dairy servings daily, and only 12% of teenage girls and 14% of women consume the recommended amounts.[a] In addition to missing out on the benefits of whole grain and fruit, we eat too much added sugar. The average American consumes about 64 pounds (29 kg) of sugar a year, or about 20 teaspoons (0.1 liters) a day of added sugar, mostly from soft drinks. Americans drink over 13 billion gallons (49 billion liters) of soda every year.[b] The typical American diet, along with a lack of physical activity, contributes to the development of chronic diseases, such as diabetes, obesity, heart disease, and cancer, which are the major causes of illness and death among the U.S. population. One estimate suggests that 14% of all premature deaths in the United States result from a poor diet and a sedentary lifestyle. Experts say the best way to reduce disease is to get more exercise and choose a diet that meets recommendations.

a   Cleveland, E., J. E. Cook, J. W. Wilson, et al. "Pyramid Servings from the 1994 CSFII data ARS Food Survey Research." Available online at *http://www.barc.usda.gov/bhnrc/foodsurveys/home.html.*

b   "Pouring Rights: Marketing Empty Calories." *Public Health Reports*, vol. 115. New York: Oxford University Press, 2000, pp. 308–319.

nutrient in the body. Water intake must equal output to maintain balance. Vitamins and minerals are needed in the diet in small amounts. They both have regulatory roles and some minerals also provide structure. Consuming too much or too little energy or nutrients results in malnutrition. The Dietary Reference Intakes (DRIs) recommend amounts of energy and nutrients needed to promote health, prevent deficiencies, and reduce the incidence of chronic disease. The Daily Values on food labels, the Food Guide Pyramid, and the Dietary Guidelines for Americans present recommendations for choosing foods that will make up a healthy diet.

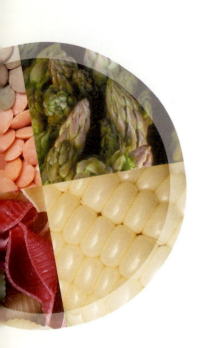

5

Balancing Intake and Output: How Many Calories Do You Need?

How many calories do you need to eat to maintain your weight? The answer depends on your age, gender, size, and activity level. To maintain your weight, the energy (calories) you consume in food must be equal to the amount your body uses to stay alive, to move, and to grow. When this occurs, your body is in energy balance and your weight will be stable, neither increasing nor decreasing (Figure 5.1). Being in energy balance, however, does not mean you are at a healthy weight. Energy intake can be in balance with energy output at any weight—fat, lean, or in between. Likewise, regardless of your current weight, if you consume more energy than you expend, the excess energy will be stored for later use, mostly as fat, and your

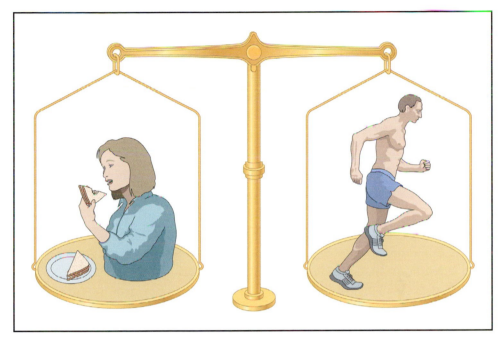

Figure 5.1 When someone is in energy balance, the amount of energy (calories) he or she consumes in food is equal to the amount of energy the body uses to function.

weight will increase. If you expend more energy than you consume, stored energy will be used to fuel your body and you will lose weight.

WHERE DOES YOUR ENERGY COME FROM?

The energy needed to fuel your body comes from the carbohydrate, fat, protein, and alcohol you consume. Vitamins, minerals, and water do not provide energy. Some of the energy you consume in food is used immediately and some is stored in your body to be used as an energy source when food is not available.

The Energy You Eat in Food

The amount of energy you consume depends on how much and what type of food you eat. In the laboratory, the amount of energy in a particular food can be measured using a **bomb calorimeter**. This device is based on the principle that energy can be converted from one form to another. To determine the energy in a food, a sample of the food is dried and placed in a chamber that is surrounded by a jacket of water. The food is then burned, converting the energy it contains into heat, and raising the temperature of the water. The increase in water temperature is then used to calculate the amount of energy in the food, based on the fact that 1 calorie is the amount of heat needed to increase the temperature of 1 kilogram (35 ounces) of water by 1°C (33.8°F).

Most of us don't have a bomb calorimeter in our kitchen, but we can still determine how much energy is in certain foods by looking at food labels or food composition tables and databases. The number of calories in a food or meal can also be estimated if you know the amounts of carbohydrate, fat, and protein that food or meal contains. Based on information gained from bomb calorimeter measurements, we know that carbohydrate and protein provide about 4 calories per gram. So for example, 5 grams of sugar, which is almost pure carbohydrate, contains about 20 calories (5 g x 4 Cal/g). We also know that fat provides 9 calories per gram, so 5 grams of corn oil, which is almost pure fat, contains about 45 calories (5 g x 9 Cal/g). Because most foods are mixtures of carbohydrate, protein, and fat, the arithmetic is a little more complicated. For example, a half-cup serving of macaroni and cheese contains 8 grams of protein, 20 grams of carbohydrate, and 11 grams of fat; its energy content is therefore:

(4 Cal/g x 8 g protein) + (4 Cal/g x 20 g carbohydrate) + (9 Cal/g x 11 g fat) = 211 Calories

The Energy You Store in Your Body

Your body stores energy as glycogen and as fat. These energy sources are stored when the amount of energy consumed in food exceeds the body's immediate needs. Glycogen is stored carbohydrate. It is made up of branching chains of glucose molecules. Glycogen is stored in your muscles and liver. Muscle glycogen is used to fuel muscle contraction. Liver glycogen is used to provide blood glucose that can be transported to cells throughout the body. Together, the glycogen in the muscles and liver provides

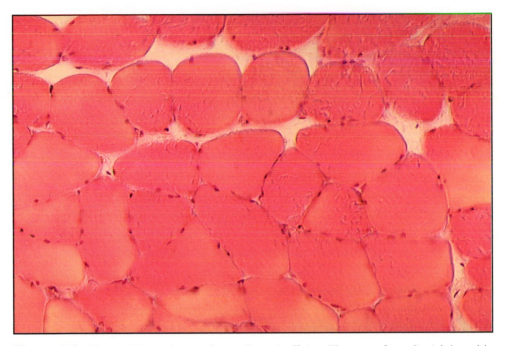

Figure 5.2 Most of the volume of an adipocyte (fat cell) comes from its triglyceride content. When we store more energy, the amount of triglycerides in each cell increases and the adipocytes (seen here) grow in size.

about 1,400 calories of stored energy. Fat stores are in the form of triglycerides. Triglycerides are made up of three fatty acids linked to a molecule of glycerol. Triglycerides are stored primarily in adipose tissue. Adipose tissue is made up of fat cells called **adipocytes**. When excess energy is consumed, triglycerides accumulate and adipocytes increase in size (Figure 5.2). Most adipocytes are formed between infancy and adolescence. In adulthood, only excessive weight gain can cause the production of new adipocytes. The greater the number of adipocytes an individual has, the greater his or her ability to store fat.

Using Your Stored Energy

What do you use for energy between meals? When energy intake does not meet energy needs, whether it is between meals or over the course of days, weeks, or months, body stores are used to supply the additional energy. Some tissues, including the brain and red blood cells, must use glucose as an energy source. Initially, this glucose is supplied by the breakdown of stored glycogen. When glycogen stores begin to decrease, such as when no food has been eaten for more than several hours, additional glucose can be synthesized by a metabolic pathway called **gluconeogenesis**. Gluconeogenesis uses small molecules derived primarily from the breakdown of amino acids as the raw material for glucose production. To obtain these amino acids, small amounts of body protein, primarily muscle protein, must be broken down. Because the body does not store protein, when it is broken down to provide amino acids for gluconeogenesis, functional body proteins are lost.

Energy for tissues that don't require glucose is provided by the breakdown of body fat. Stored triglycerides are broken into glycerol and fatty acids, which can be metabolized to produce energy. However, a small amount of glucose is needed to completely break down fatty acids. When glucose is limited, the incomplete breakdown of fatty acids produces **ketones**. These ketones can be used as an energy source by many tissues; during starvation, even the brain can adapt to use ketones to supply some of its energy needs. This reduces the amount of glucose needed and, therefore, decreases the amount of protein that is broken down to provide glucose. Ketone production is a normal adaptation to starvation, but if large amounts of ketones are produced, as occurs in diabetes, they build up in the blood, resulting in a condition called **ketosis**. Ketosis changes the acidity of the blood and can eventually result in coma and death.

When meals are eaten every few hours, some of the energy in glycogen and fat stores is used between meals and replaced by energy consumed in the next meal so that there is no net change in the amount of stored energy. However, if energy stores are not replenished, the amount of stored energy—and hence, body weight—will decrease. It is estimated that an energy deficit of about 3,500 calories results in the loss of a pound (0.45 kg) of fat.

Adding to Your Energy Stores

The energy we consume in meals and snacks throughout the day is often more than is needed by our bodies at that moment in time. The body must therefore determine which nutrients it will use immediately and which it will store for later. This determination is based on what the body needs, which nutrients can be stored, and how efficiently they can be stored. When alcohol is consumed, it is quickly broken down and used for energy. This is because it is toxic and the body cannot store it. When protein is consumed, its constituent amino acids are used to synthesize body proteins and other nitrogen-containing molecules. Then, any excess amino acids are broken down and used for energy. When carbohydrate is consumed, it is used to supply blood glucose and to build glycogen stores. Once glycogen stores are full, the remaining carbohydrate is used for energy. When fat is consumed, it is used to meet immediate energy needs and any remaining dietary fat is stored as triglycerides, primarily in adipose tissue.

Most of the fat deposited in adipose tissue comes from dietary fat. This is because excess fat is readily stored and the energy required to convert dietary fat to stored body fat is very small. Fat can be stored in the body in virtually unlimited amounts. It is not needed to build tissues as proteins are or to provide blood glucose as carbohydrates are. Dietary fat consumed in excess of needs can be transported directly to the adipose tissue. At the adipose tissue, an enzyme on the surface of cells lining the blood vessels breaks the triglycerides into fatty acids and glycerol, which can then enter the adipocytes. These are then reassembled into triglycerides for storage. The body is capable of converting excess carbohydrate and amino acids into fat for storage. However, under normal dietary circumstances, this doesn't occur because it involves numerous metabolic reactions and the body must expend energy in the conversion process.

WHAT DO WE USE ENERGY FOR?

The total amount of energy used by the body each day is called **total energy expenditure**. Total energy expenditure includes the energy needed to maintain basal functions, process food, and fuel physical activity. During growth and pregnancy, total energy expenditure also includes the energy used to deposit new tissues. During lactation, it includes the energy used to produce milk. There is also a small amount of energy used to maintain body temperature in a cold environment.

Energy to Stay Alive

The portion of the energy requirement used for basic body functions such as breathing, circulating blood, and maintaining a constant body temperature is referred to as **basal energy expenditure**. Basal energy expenditure accounts for about 60 to 75% of the body's total energy requirement. It is defined as the minimum amount of energy needed to keep an awake, resting body alive. Basal energy expenditure includes the energy necessary for all metabolic reactions and life-sustaining functions, but it does not include the energy needed for the digestion and absorption of food or for physical activity. The rate at which energy is used to keep the body alive is called **basal metabolic rate** (**BMR**); it is usually expressed in calories per hour. In order to measure the energy that is needed for basal functions, energy expenditure must be measured in a warm room, in the morning before rising, and at least 12 hours after food intake or activity. Measurements done in this way minimize any residual energy expenditure from activity or digestion and absorption. Because of the difficulty of achieving the conditions needed for BMR measurements, energy expenditure is often measured after only five to six hours without food or exercise. These measures yield values referred to as **resting energy expenditure** or **resting metabolic rate** (**RMR**). RMR values are about 10 to 20% higher than BMR.

Basal needs are affected by body weight, the amount of **lean body mass**, gender, age, and growth rate. Needs increase with increasing body weight; BMR is higher in heavier individuals. The amount of lean body mass also affects needs because it requires more energy to maintain lean tissue than it does to maintain fat; basal needs are generally higher in individuals who have more lean tissue. Men typically have higher energy needs than women because they have greater lean body mass. Basal needs are lower in older adults, partly due to a decrease in lean body mass that occurs with age. Basal needs are increased during periods of rapid growth because energy is required to produce new body tissue.

Basal energy needs can be affected by certain abnormal conditions. An elevation in body temperature, such as that which occurs when you have a fever, increases energy needs. It is estimated that for every 1°F (-17°C) above normal body temperature, there is a 7% increase in RMR. Surgery and injury can increase needs because energy is required to repair body tissues. Abnormal levels of thyroid hormones can also affect basal needs. An overproduction of thyroid hormones, called hyperthyroidism, increases energy needs, whereas hypothyroidism, an underproduction of thyroid hormones, decreases energy needs and can lead to weight gain. The effect of thyroid hormones on energy needs and body weight is the reason obesity was once explained as a glandular problem. It is now known that obesity due to a lack of thyroid hormone is rare.

Energy needs may also be affected by consuming insufficient energy. Consuming a low-calorie diet for a long period of time may depress metabolic rate as the body attempts to conserve energy. This drop in BMR decreases the amount of energy needed to maintain weight. This is a beneficial adaptation in starvation, but it makes intentional weight loss more difficult.

Energy to Process Your Food

You get energy from food, but you need energy to digest food and to absorb, metabolize, and store the nutrients from this food. This energy expenditure is called the **thermic effect of food** (**TEF**), or **diet-induced thermogenesis**. It causes body temperature to rise slightly for several hours after eating. TEF is estimated to be about 10% of energy intake but can vary depending on the amounts and types of nutrients consumed. TEF increases with the size of the meal because it takes energy to store the excess nutrients. A meal that is high in fat has a lower TEF than a meal high in carbohydrate or protein because fat is stored more efficiently. This difference in the energy cost of storing energy from fat, carbohydrate, and protein means a diet high in fat may produce more body fat than a diet high in carbohydrate.

Energy to Keep You Moving

Physical activity, whether it involves standing and talking on the telephone or running a marathon, requires energy above that needed for basal needs. In most cases, activity accounts for 15 to 30% of total energy expenditure, but this varies greatly depending on how much activity is performed and how strenuous it is. For example, a construction worker who spends many hours a day doing physical labor uses a great deal more energy in daily activities than does an office worker who spends most of the day sitting at a desk. It takes more energy to jog for 30 minutes than it does to walk for 30 minutes, but if you walk for an hour you will expend about as much as if you jogged for 30 minutes. Energy expenditure is also affected by body size. Because it takes more energy to move a heavier object, the amount of energy expended for many activities increases as body weight increases (Table 5.1).

MEASURING HOW MUCH ENERGY IS USED

To be in energy balance, the amount of energy consumed must equal the amount of energy used by the body. Scientists have developed a number of ways to measure how much energy a person uses. **Direct calorimetry** assesses energy expenditure by measuring heat production. In humans, direct calorimetry measures the amount of heat given off by the body. This heat is generated by metabolic reactions that both convert food energy into ATP and use ATP for body processes. The heat produced is proportional to the amount of energy

---

FACT BOX 5.1

Exercise Extremes

The number of calories we burn during exercise varies greatly from person to person. Many people burn only a few hundred calories each day through exercise, but for others the numbers are extreme. The average rider in the Tour de France bicycle race burns 6,000–7,000 calories each day during the 3-week race and may burn over 10,000 calories on the days he or she rides 120 miles (193 km) through the mountains.

Table 5.1 Calories Burned for Various Activities

ACTIVITY	ENERGY (CAL/HR)						
BODY WEIGHT (LB)	110	125	140	155	170	185	200
Sitting							
Male	73	77	81	85	89	93	97
Female	63	66	69	72	76	79	82
Bowling							
Male	121	128	135	142	148	155	162
Female	105	110	115	121	126	131	136
Aerobics							
Male	455	480	506	531	556	582	607
Female	394	413	433	453	472	492	511
Biking (12 mph)							
Male	380	401	422	443	464	486	507
Female	329	345	361	378	394	410	427
Walking (15 min/mi)							
Male	257	271	285	300	314	328	342
Female	222	233	244	255	266	277	288
Gardening							
Male	303	320	337	354	371	388	405
Female	263	276	289	302	315	328	341
Weight lifting							
Male	340	359	378	397	415	434	453
Female	294	309	323	338	352	367	382
Swimming (laps)							
Male	364	384	405	425	445	465	486
Female	315	331	346	362	378	393	409
Dancing							
Male	364	384	405	425	445	465	486
Female	315	331	346	362	378	393	409
Golf (walking w/bag)							
Male	425	448	472	496	519	543	567
Female	368	386	404	422	441	459	477
Jumping rope							
Male	595	628	661	694	727	760	793
Female	515	540	566	591	617	642	668
Running (10 min/mi)							
Male	619	653	688	722	757	791	826
Female	536	562	589	615	642	669	695

used by the individual. Direct calorimetry is an accurate method for measuring energy expenditure, but it is expensive and impractical because it requires that the person being assessed remain in an insulated chamber throughout the evaluation.

A less cumbersome method of estimating energy expenditure is **indirect calorimetry**, which estimates energy use by assessing nutrient utilization. It measures the amounts of oxygen consumed and carbon dioxide expired by the body. The body's energy use can be calculated from these values because the burning of fuels by the body in cellular respiration uses oxygen and produces carbon dioxide. Oxygen use and carbon dioxide production can be measured by analyzing the difference between inhaled and exhaled air. Measuring the composition of respired gases requires that you breathe into a mask or ventilated hood. Indirect calorimetry can be used to measure the energy used for individual components of expenditure, such as physical activity or RMR. It can also be used to estimate total energy needs, but it is not practical for measuring energy expenditure in free-living individuals because the equipment is uncomfortable and inappropriate for long-term use.

A method that can assess energy use over longer periods of time is the **doubly-labeled water method**. This method determines oxygen use and carbon dioxide production but does not require the individual to wear a mask or hood. Instead, it involves having the person ingest or be injected with water labeled with **isotopes** of oxygen and hydrogen. The labeled oxygen and hydrogen are used by the body in metabolism. By measuring the rate at which labeled oxygen and labeled hydrogen disappear from body fluids, the amount of carbon dioxide produced by the energy-requiring reactions in the body can be estimated. This method does not require the individual to carry any equipment and can be used to measure expenditure in free-living subjects for periods of up to two weeks. Doubly-labeled water is the preferred method for determining the total daily energy expenditures of both healthy and clinical populations.[21] However, it is not helpful in determining the proportions of total energy expenditure that is used for basal energy expenditure, TEF, or physical activity.

WHAT'S YOUR EER?

The current recommendations for energy intake in the United States are the **estimated energy requirements** (EER) established by the DRIs. An EER is the amount of energy predicted to maintain energy balance in a healthy person of a defined age, gender, weight, height, and level of physical activity. These values were determined from studies that used doubly-labeled water to measure energy expenditure. Equations developed from this data can be used to calculate your individual EER.

Estimating Your Physical Activity Level

In order to calculate your EER, it is necessary to estimate how active you are. By keeping a daily log of your activities and recording the amount of time you spend doing each, you can use Table 5.2 and Table 5.3 to estimate your activity level. The EER calculations use four different activity levels to estimate energy needs: sedentary, low active, active, and very active. A "sedentary" individual is one who does not participate in any activity beyond that required for daily independent living, such as housework, homework, yard work, gardening, and walking the dog. To be in the "low active" category,

---

FACT BOX 5.2

How Much Exercise Do You Get?

Americans need to move more. Over 60% of U.S. adults do not meet exercise recommendations and about 25% admit they are not active at all.[a] Women are less active than men, older people are less active than younger ones, African Americans and Hispanics are less active than whites, and less affluent people are less active than the affluent. Adults are not the only ones who need to get off the couch. Nearly half of young Americans between the ages of 12 and 21 are not vigorously active on a regular basis. About 14% of young people report no recent physical activity at all. Participation in all types of physical activity declines strikingly as age or grade in school increases.

a CDC, Physical Activity and Health. "A Report of the Surgeon General, Fact Sheets." Available online at *http://www.cdc.gov/nccdphp/sgr/fact.htm*.

Table 5.2 Intensity of Various Activities

ACTIVITIES OF DAILY LIVING	MODERATE ACTIVITIES	VIGOROUS ACTIVITIES
Gardening (no lifting)	Calisthenics (light, no weights)	Aerobics (moderate to heavy)
Watering plants	Cycling (leisurely, 6 – 7 mph)	Ballet
Raking leaves	Golf (without cart)	Climbing (hills or mountains)
Mowing the lawn	Swimming (slow)	Cycling (moderate or higher, greater than 10 mph)
Household tasks	Walking (3 mph, 20 min/mile)	
Mopping	Walking (4 mph, 15 min/mile)	Dancing (square dancing or fast ballroom)
Vacuuming		Ice skating
Walking from the house to car or bus		Jogging (12 min/mile or faster)
		Roller skating
Loading/unloading the car		Rope jumping
Walking the dog		Skiing (water, downhill, or cross country)
		Squash
		Swimming (moderate to fast)
		Tennis
		Walking (5 mph, 12 min/mile)
It is assumed that we spend about 2.5 hours per day in these types of activities.	Any activities that expend about 250 to 350 Cal/hr for a 150-lb (68-kg) individual.	Any activities that expend more than 350 Cal/hr for a 150-lb (68-kg) individual.

an adult weighing 70 kg (154 pounds) would need to expend an amount of energy equivalent to walking 2.2 miles (3.5 km) at a rate of 3 to 4 miles (4.8 to 6.4 km) per hour in addition to the activities of daily living. To be "active," this adult would need to perform daily exercise equivalent to walking 7 miles (11 km) at a rate of 3 to 4 miles (4.8 to 6.4 km) per hour, and to be "very active," he or she would

Table 5.3 Levels of Physical Activity with PA Values

PHYSICAL ACTIVITY LEVEL	PA Values			
	3–18 years		≥ 19 years	
	Boys	Girls	Men	Women
SEDENTARY: Engages in only the activities of daily living and no moderate or vigorous activities	1.00	1.00	1.00	1.00
LOW ACTIVE: Daily activity equivalent of at least 30 minutes of moderate activity and a minimum of 15 to 30 minutes of vigorous activity, depending on the intensity of the activity	1.13	1.16	1.11	1.12
ACTIVE: Engages in at least 60 minutes of moderate activity or a minimum of 30 to 60 minutes of vigorous activity, depending on the intensity of the activity	1.26	1.31	1.25	1.27
VERY ACTIVE: Engages in at least 2.5 hours of moderate activity or a minimum of 1 to 1.75 hours of vigorous activity, depending on the intensity of the activity	1.42	1.56	1.48	1.45

need to perform the equivalent of walking 17 miles (27 km) at this rate in addition to the activities of daily living. Each physical activity level is assigned a numerical **Physical Activity (PA) value** that can then be used to calculate EER.

Calculating Your EER

EER calculations take into account your age, gender, height, weight, life stage, and level of physical activity (Table 5.4). To determine your EER, enter your age in years, height in meters, weight in kilograms,

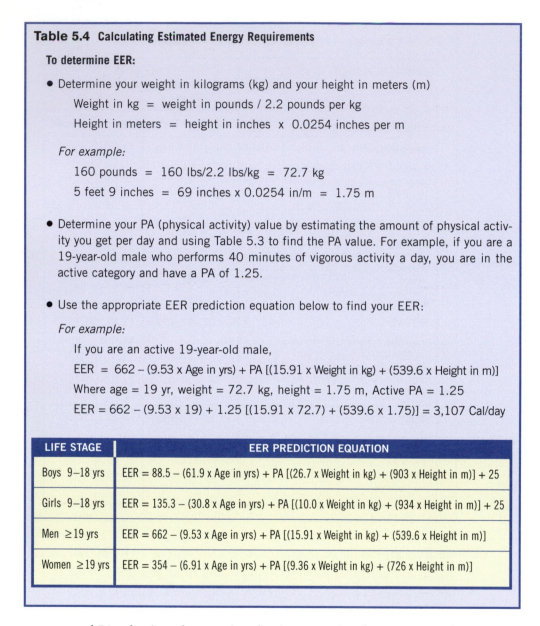

Table 5.4 Calculating Estimated Energy Requirements

To determine EER:

- Determine your weight in kilograms (kg) and your height in meters (m)

    Weight in kg = weight in pounds / 2.2 pounds per kg

    Height in meters = height in inches x 0.0254 inches per m

For example:

    160 pounds = 160 lbs/2.2 lbs/kg = 72.7 kg

    5 feet 9 inches = 69 inches x 0.0254 in/m = 1.75 m

- Determine your PA (physical activity) value by estimating the amount of physical activity you get per day and using Table 5.3 to find the PA value. For example, if you are a 19-year-old male who performs 40 minutes of vigorous activity a day, you are in the active category and have a PA of 1.25.

- Use the appropriate EER prediction equation below to find your EER:

For example:

    If you are an active 19-year-old male,

    EER = 662 − (9.53 x Age in yrs) + PA [(15.91 x Weight in kg) + (539.6 x Height in m)]

    Where age = 19 yr, weight = 72.7 kg, height = 1.75 m, Active PA = 1.25

    EER = 662 − (9.53 x 19) + 1.25 [(15.91 x 72.7) + (539.6 x 1.75)] = 3,107 Cal/day

LIFE STAGE	EER PREDICTION EQUATION
Boys 9–18 yrs	EER = 88.5 − (61.9 x Age in yrs) + PA [(26.7 x Weight in kg) + (903 x Height in m)] + 25
Girls 9–18 yrs	EER = 135.3 − (30.8 x Age in yrs) + PA [(10.0 x Weight in kg) + (934 x Height in m)] + 25
Men ≥19 yrs	EER = 662 − (9.53 x Age in yrs) + PA [(15.91 x Weight in kg) + (539.6 x Height in m)]
Women ≥19 yrs	EER = 354 − (6.91 x Age in yrs) + PA [(9.36 x Weight in kg) + (726 x Height in m)]

and PA value into the equation that is appropriate for your age and gender. The EER values for infants, children, and adolescents include the energy used to deposit tissues associated with growth. Beginning at age three, there are separate EER equations for boys and girls because of differences in growth and physical activity. The EER for pregnancy is determined as the sum of the total energy expenditure of a nonpregnant woman plus the energy needed to maintain pregnancy and deposit maternal and fetal tissue. During lactation, EER is the sum of the total energy expenditure of nonlactating women and the energy in the milk produced, minus the energy mobilized from maternal tissue stores.

Activity level has a significant effect on EER. For example, a 30-year-old woman who is 5 feet 5 inches (1.65 m) tall and weighs 130 pounds (59 kg) has an EER of about 1,900 Cal/day if she is sedentary. If she increases her activity to the "active" level, her EER increases to 2,370 Cal/day. In order to maintain a healthy weight and reduce the risk of chronic disease, physical activity at the "active" level is recommended.

CONNECTIONS

When body weight is stable, the number of calories you consume is equal to the number expended, and you are in energy balance. The energy used to fuel the body comes from the food you eat and energy stores in the body. Protein, carbohydrate, fat, and alcohol in your diet provide energy (calories). Energy is stored in the body as glycogen and triglycerides. When you eat food, some of the energy is used for immediate needs and the rest is stored. These stores are then used when you have not eaten for a few hours or for longer. Fat is the nutrient that is most efficiently stored in the body; it can be stored in virtually limitless quantities in the adipocytes. The body uses energy to maintain basal functions such as the beating of the heart, to digest and absorb nutrients, and to fuel activity. The amount of energy used in activity is affected by how much exercise you get. The amount of energy needed by the body can be measured in a number of ways—the best method for long-term measurements is the doubly-labeled water technique. Individual energy needs can be estimated by calculating EER from standard equations.

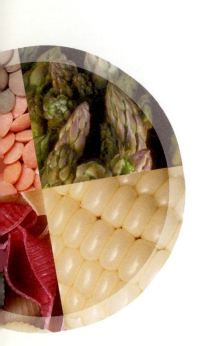

6

Biological Factors That Affect What You Weigh

The principle of energy balance tells us that if you eat the same number of calories you use, your weight will remain the same. But have you ever known someone who can eat whatever he or she wants without gaining an ounce? Or someone who seems to eat very little but is overweight? This can be explained by the fact that body weight and fat are regulated to remain at a particular level in each person. This level is influenced by your genes.

GENES AND BODY WEIGHT

In most people, body fat and weight remain remarkably constant over long periods despite fluctuations in food intake and activity level. This is extraordinary, considering how variable most people's food intake is from day to day. The signals that regulate body weight, body size, body shape, and the amount of body fat are carried in your genes.

Our understanding of how a person's genetic background contributes to body fatness is expanding rapidly. Thus far, a host of genes involved in the regulation of body weight have been identified in rodents, and similar genes have been found in humans.[22] These genes are often referred to as "obesity genes." The proteins made by obesity genes are often involved in sending signals about energy intake and levels of body fat stores to the brain. Most human obesity is not likely to be due to a single abnormal gene but rather to variations in many genes that interact with one another and the environment to regulate body shape and size as well as energy intake and expenditure.

HOW IS BODY WEIGHT REGULATED?

Body weight is regulated by matching energy intake to energy output. If intake increases, expenditure must also increase to prevent weight gain. There are two types of regulatory systems that modulate energy intake and expenditure to keep body weight at a set level. One type is concerned with short-term weight regulation. It regulates how much and how often you eat on any given day. The other is concerned with longer-term regulation and is involved in monitoring and responding to the amount of body fat you have over the long run. Some of these short-term and long-term regulatory mechanisms act through the release of hormones. These hormones travel in the blood and then act in a region of the brain called the **hypothalamus**, where they trigger short-term and long-term changes in appetite and metabolism.

Short-term Regulation: Are You Hungry or Full?

How much you eat for breakfast and when you get hungry for dinner are, to some extent, determined by short-term regulatory mechanisms that affect hunger and **satiety**. The physiological sensations of hunger and satiety are the result of internal signals that come from the gastrointestinal tract, circulating nutrients, or signals from the brain.[23] Some of these signals are due to the presence or absence of food in the gastrointestinal tract. The simplest type of signal about food intake comes from local nerves in the walls of the stomach and small intestine that sense the volume or pressure of food and send a message to the brain to either start or stop food intake. The presence of glucose, fat, and amino acids in the gastrointestinal tract also sends information directly to the brain and triggers the release of gastrointestinal hormones that promote satiety.[24] Absorbed nutrients may also send information to the brain to modulate food intake. Circulating levels of nutrients, including glucose, amino acids, ketones, and fatty acids, are monitored by the brain and may trigger signals to eat or not to eat.[25] Nutrients that are taken up by the brain may affect **neurotransmitter** concentrations, which then affect the amount and type of nutrients consumed. For example, some studies suggest that when levels of the neurotransmitter serotonin in the brain are low, carbohydrate is craved, but when they are high, protein is preferred.[25] The liver may also be involved in signaling hunger and satiety. Absorbed water-soluble nutrients go directly to the liver, where they affect liver metabolism. Changes in liver metabolism, in particular the amount of ATP, are believed to modulate food intake.[22]

Hormones released before and after eating also help regulate when we eat meals and how much we eat. The hormone insulin is released by the pancreas in response to the intake of carbohydrate and allows the uptake of glucose by cells. It may affect hunger and satiety by lowering the levels of circulating nutrients. The hormone **ghrelin**, produced by the stomach, is believed to stimulate your desire to eat meals at usual times. For example, you typically feel hungry around lunchtime regardless of when and how much you had for breakfast. Ghrelin levels have been found to rise an hour or two before a meal and drop very low after a meal. Overproduction of ghrelin could contribute to obesity because levels have been found to increase in people who have lost weight through dieting, so it may be a part of what undermines the ability to keep weight off.[26] Peptide PYY is a hormone that causes a reduction in appetite and food intake. It is released from the gastrointestinal tract after a meal and the amount released is proportional to the calorie content of the meal.[27]

The Long Term: Regulating How Much Body Fat You Have

Most of us overeat on occasion—for example, at a birthday party or on summer vacation. We also under eat—some days we are too busy to stop for lunch or we feel too hot to cook dinner. These highs and lows of intake rarely result in long-term weight changes. The reason for this is that the body is able to monitor its level of body fat and prevent long-term changes in energy balance that affect weight.

Some of the information about how much fat we store comes from hormones, such as insulin and **leptin**, that are secreted in proportion to the amount of body fat.[24] Insulin is secreted from the pancreas when blood glucose levels rise; its circulating concentration is proportional to the amount of body fat. Insulin can affect food intake and body weight by sending signals to the brain and by affecting the amount of leptin produced and secreted.[23] In the brain, insulin has an appetite-suppressing effect; however, the effect of insulin in the brain is not as great as that of leptin. Leptin is produced by the adipocytes and the amount of leptin produced is proportional to the size of adipocytes, so more leptin is released as fat stores grow. When leptin levels are high, mechanisms that cause an increase in energy expenditure and a decrease in food intake are stimulated, and pathways that promote food intake, and hence, weight gain, are inhibited. When fat stores shrink, less leptin is released. Low leptin levels in the brain allow pathways that decrease energy expenditure and increase food intake to become active. Thus, leptin acts like a thermostat to keep body fatness from changing (Figure 6.1).[25]

DEFECTS IN REGULATION: A CAUSE OF OBESITY?

If someone is born with a defective leptin gene, leptin is not produced normally and the person will become obese. When leptin was first discovered, there was hope that scientists had found both the cause and the cure for obesity. Although a few cases of obesity due to a mutation in the leptin gene have been identified, mutations in this gene are not responsible for most human obesity. Rather, most human obesity is likely to be due to a combination of genes that contribute to excessive food intake or reductions in energy

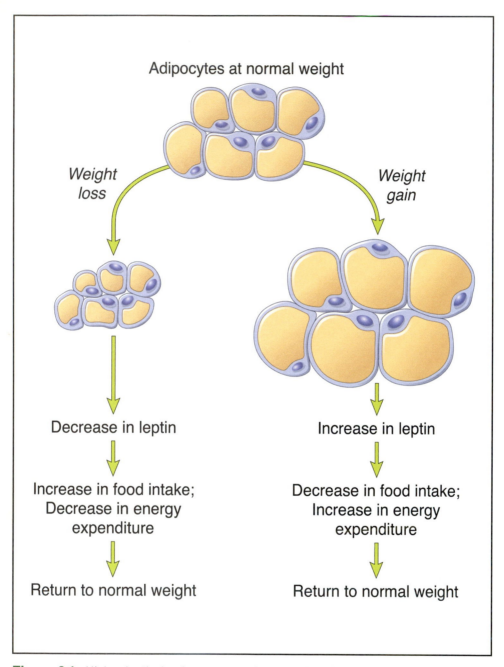

Figure 6.1 Higher leptin levels cause people to eat less food and expend more energy. When leptin levels fall, people eat more and use less energy.

output. Reductions in energy output may be due to abnormalities in basal metabolism, the ability to burn off extra calories, or the amount of energy expended in physical activity.

Do Obese People Have a Slower Metabolism?

Many overweight people contend that they eat very few calories and still continue to gain weight. This would imply that their energy expenditure is less than in normal-weight individuals. One possible explanation for this is that overweight individuals inherit a thrifty metabolism. An individual with a thrifty metabolism theoretically uses energy very efficiently so that more of the energy consumed is converted into ATP or deposited in energy stores than in someone with a less efficient metabolism. This person would therefore need to

---

FACT BOX 6.1

We Evolved to Store Fat—Not to Lose It

Humans appear to be better at protecting against weight loss than defending against weight gain. Evidence for this is found in the way the hormone leptin works. When fat cells shrink and less leptin is released, we eat more and use less energy to help us maintain or regain body fat. However, when fat cells expand and leptin levels rise, we eat less and expend more energy. Beyond a certain level, an increase in leptin has little effect. This is illustrated by the fact that obese people generally have high leptin levels in the blood, but these high levels don't help them lose weight.[a] Leptin appears to have evolved to protect us against famine rather than against weight gain when food is plentiful. When referring to the fact that humans are better at gaining weight than at losing it, Rudolph Leibel, a geneticist at Columbia University College of Physicians and Surgeons, says, "you can bemoan the fact that we're set up this way, but it's what's gotten us here." It is, after all, our ability to store and preserve body fat that has helped the human race to survive the famines that have plagued us throughout history.

a Considine, R. V., M. K. Sinha, M. L. Heinman, et al. "Serum immunoreactive-leptin concentrations in normal weight and obese humans." *New England Journal of Medicine* 334 (1996): 292–295.

eat less to maintain a particular body weight. But actual studies of energy intake in overweight individuals have been inconclusive, in part because determining energy intake is difficult; there is evidence that overweight individuals are more likely to underreport their energy intake than their lean counterparts.[28] Studies using doubly-labeled water have shown that energy expenditure increases with increasing body weight, suggesting that obese individuals need to eat more rather than less than lean controls to maintain their higher body weight. Although some people may need fewer calories than others, there is little evidence that a thrifty metabolism is a factor in the majority of human obesity.

Can Obese People Burn off Extra Calories?

The regulation of energy expenditure in response to changes in circumstance such as trauma, changes in temperature, and changes in food intake is referred to as **adaptive thermogenesis**. Increased energy expenditure through adaptive thermogenesis may prevent some of the weight gain that accompanies an increase in energy intake.[29] When body weight is increased above normal by overeating, energy expenditure increases to burn extra calories and return weight to the original level. Likewise, in experiments in which food intake is restricted and people lose weight, energy expenditure decreases to prevent weight loss. These responses occur in both obese and lean people, but some studies have found that the drop in energy expenditure seen with weight reduction was greater in obese subjects than in lean subjects, and the increase in energy expenditure seen with weight gain was less in obese subjects than in lean subjects.[28] This difference in the adaptive responses in energy expenditure between lean and obese subjects may be one reason why it is so hard for obese people to keep weight off.

Several biochemical mechanisms have been proposed to explain adaptive thermogenesis. The first is substrate cycling, or futile cycling, which wastes energy by allowing opposing biochemical reactions to occur simultaneously. For example, a molecule is formed and then broken down; the result is that energy is consumed but there is no net change in the number of molecules in the body, and therefore, no storage of energy as fat. A second way that excess energy might be used is by separating or uncoupling the **electron transport chain** from the production of ATP. When this occurs, energy is lost as heat rather than being converted to a form that can be used by the body. Several proteins that uncouple the electron transport chain from the

---

FACT BOX 6.2

Why Are Most Pima Indians Fat?

An example of human obesity that clearly demonstrates the interaction of genes and environment is the Pima Indian population living in Arizona. More than 75% of this group of Pimas is obese. Scientists have identified a number of genes that may be responsible for this group's tendency to store more body fat.[a] Typically, Pimas have lower than average energy needs. This is a good trait when it comes to survival during times of shortage, but it becomes a negative trait when food is plentiful and the workload is light. Today's Pimas get little exercise in their daily lives and they have abandoned the traditional diet eaten by their ancestors in favor of the high-fat, high-calorie diet typical in the rest of the United States. Together, their genetic makeup, their activity level, and their food intake have led them to have high levels of body fat. In contrast to Pimas in the United States, there is a group of Pima Indians living in Mexico who have a much lower rate of obesity. They have the same genes as the Pimas in the United States, but they are farmers who eat the food they grow and have a high level of physical activity.[b] Despite their diet and exercise patterns, they still have higher rates of obesity, which shows that their genes favor high body weight. However, they are significantly less obese than the Arizona Pima Indians are. These two Pima populations clearly show the interactions between heredity and environment in determining body weight.

a Norman, R. A., D. B. Thompson, T. Foroud, et al, "Genomewide search for genes influencing percent body fact in Pima Indians: Suggestive linkage at chromosome 11q21–q22." *American Journal of Human Genetics* 60 (1997): 166–173.

b Esparza, J., C. Fox, I. T. Harper, et al. "Daily energy expenditure in Mexican and USA Pima Indians: Low physical activity as a possible cause of obesity." *International Journal of Obesity and Related Metabolic Disorders* 24 (2000): 55–59.

production of ATP have been identified in human muscle, white adipose tissue, lung, spleen, white blood cells, bone marrow, and stomach.[30] It is hypothesized that these proteins may be involved in increasing energy output to regulate body weight in humans.

Do Obese People Fidget Less?

The amount of energy an individual expends depends primarily on metabolic rate and activity level. Genetics determine our metabolic rate. Activity level is affected by genetics and individual choices. Individuals with more body fat tend to exercise less, but the amount of voluntary exercise we get may not be the only type of activity that contributes to energy expenditure. Energy is also expended in involuntary exercise, such as fidgeting, maintenance of posture, and the other small movements that occur during daily living. A study of overfed nonobese individuals found that there was a tenfold variation in the amount of fat gained. Some subjects were able to increase energy expenditure to a greater extent and so gained less fat. Some of the differences in weight gain may have been due to differences in adaptive thermogenesis, but about two-thirds of the increase in energy expenditure that occurred with overfeeding was found to be due to an increase in involuntary exercise.[31] Individuals who gained

FACT BOX 6.3

Fidgeting the Fat Away

When different people overeat by the same amount, some gain more weight than others. A study was done to test how involuntary movements such as fidgeting, spontaneous muscle contraction, and moving to maintain posture may help prevent weight gain. The study found a large variation between individuals. People in the study ate an extra 1,000 calories a day. Some showed no increase in involuntary movement, whereas others moved and fidgeted a lot more—burning as much as 692 calories a day—the equivalent of a 180-pound (82-kg) man jogging for an hour!

Source: Levine, J. A., N. L. Eberhardt, and M. D. Jensen. "Role of nonexercise activity thermogenesis in resistance to fat gain in humans." *Science* 283 (1999): 212–214.

little weight had a greater level of involuntary exercise than those who gained more weight. It is still not known what mechanisms control why some people respond to excess energy by becoming restless and fidgeting more while others remain lethargic in their daily activities.

CONNECTIONS

The signals that regulate body size, body shape, body weight, and body fat are carried in our genes. Genes that affect body weight are referred to as obesity genes. These genes make proteins that relay messages about how much we eat and how much energy we expend. Body weight is regulated in the short term by mechanisms that affect hunger and satiety and therefore how much and how often we eat during the day. Other regulators of body weight, such as the hormone leptin, work over the long term by monitoring the amount of body fat. Some human obesity may be due to a combination of genes that result in a lower than normal energy expenditure or an inability to increase energy expenditure to compensate for an increase in intake. Factors that may contribute to obesity in some people include a slow metabolism that allows them to eat little but maintain their weight, a reduced ability to burn off extra calories when they are consumed, and a lower amount of involuntary activity when excess energy is consumed.

7

Achieving and Maintaining a Healthy Weight

Managing your weight to keep it in the healthy range will help you stay healthy. The health problems associated with obesity and the alarming failure rate of long-term weight loss have caused researchers and physicians to reevaluate the way they think about this problem. They now suggest that weight problems should be viewed in terms of weight management. Managing weight is important for everyone, whether individuals are at a healthy weight or not. For those at a healthy weight, the goal of weight management is to keep their weight in the healthy range. For those who are already overweight, the goal of weight management is to reduce body fat to a healthy level that can be maintained over a lifetime or, at a minimum, to prevent further weight gain.[32] Reducing energy intake, increasing activity, and changing behaviors that contribute to weight gain can help individuals achieve and maintain a healthy weight.

WHO NEEDS TO LOSE WEIGHT?

The first step in managing weight is assessment. An evaluation of current weight and weight history, along with a review of medical conditions, can help determine whether or not weight loss is recommended. Whether or not you are overweight can be established by determining your BMI. In general, a BMI above the healthy range means that weight loss would improve long-term health, but this is not always the case. Some people with high BMIs, such as weight lifters, may have a greater muscle mass but not more body fat than is recommended. If, in addition to a high BMI, body fat is elevated or waist circumference is increased, weight loss is usually recommended. Age is also important because extra weight may be less of a health risk at certain times in life. For example, for a teen who is still growing, an increase in body weight may be followed by a growth spurt that puts BMI back in the healthy range. In older adults, a few extra pounds may provide a reserve in the event of a long-term illness.

A key factor in whether or not weight loss is recommended is the presence of diseases and abnormalities associated with excess body fat (Table 7.1). For example, blood pressure, blood sugar, and blood cholesterol levels all increase with body weight and with them the risk of heart disease and diabetes. If someone is overweight and has two or more of these conditions, weight loss is recommended. A family history of these conditions is also a consideration in determining whether or not weight loss is necessary to promote health. Based on these criteria, not everyone who is a few pounds over ideal body weight should lose the extra weight. People with no health conditions associated with excess body fat and who have a healthy lifestyle but have a BMI in the overweight range (25–29.9) may not benefit from weight loss. For example, a person with a BMI of 28 whose blood pressure and cholesterol are normal and who exercises regularly would not reduce his or her health risks by losing weight. For such a person, weight management may mean simply preventing further weight gain. For others, this risk assessment may indicate that body weight is a health risk and a weight loss plan should be developed. For example, for a person with a BMI of 28 who has high blood pressure and high blood cholesterol levels, weight loss would be recommended to stay healthy.

Table 7.1—Conditions That Increase the Risk of Excess Weight

Cardiovascular Disease
- Blood pressure increases as body weight increases
- Total cholesterol increases as body weight increases
- Triglycerides increase as body weight increases
- LDL cholesterol increases as body weight increases
- HDL cholesterol falls as body weight increases

Type 2 Diabetes
- Fasting blood sugar increases with increasing body weight
- 80% of people with type 2 diabetes are obese
- BMI >35 increases risk by as much as 30-fold

Respiratory Problems
- Sleep apnea is more common in overweight people
- Being overweight increases the muscular work of breathing
- Asthma is worse at increased weight

Gallbladder disease is more common in overweight people

Osteoarthritis and **degenerative joint diseases** are more prevalent with increasing weight

Menstrual irregularities are increased in overweight women

Cancer
- Obese women are at increased risk for cancers of the endometrium, breast, cervix, and ovaries
- Obese men are at increased risk for colorectal and prostate cancer

Physical Inactivity
- Obese individuals who are inactive have higher risks of illness and death
- Inactivity increases the likelihood of developing diabetes and heart disease

Most obese people have tried repeatedly to lose weight. Although many succeed in the short term, most people gain back the weight they have lost within a year or two. Repeated cycles of weight loss and regain are referred to as weight cycling (Figure 7.1). **Weight cycling** increases the proportion of body fat with each successive weight regain and causes a decrease in basal metabolic rate (the rate at which

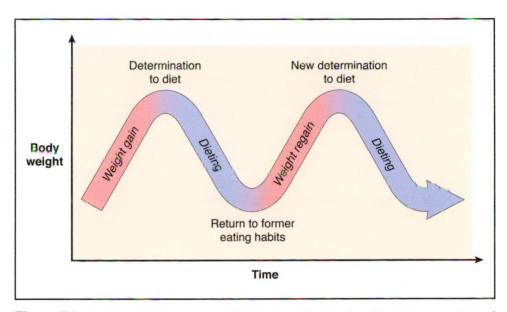

Figure 7.1 Rapid weight loss is more likely to be gained back—this causes a pattern of weight cycling. Each time the weight is regained, it becomes harder to lose.

that person uses calories), making subsequent weight loss more difficult. Despite this, weight loss is still recommended in an individual who has lost and regained weight in the past if that individual is still obese or overweight and has two or more health conditions that are associated with obesity.

HOW MUCH WEIGHT SHOULD YOU LOSE?

The medical goal for weight loss in an overweight person is to reduce the health risks associated with being overweight. The initial goal of weight loss should be to reduce body weight by approximately 10% over a period of about 6 months.[12] After this initial weight loss, risks can be reassessed to determine if additional weight loss would be beneficial.

How Fast Should You Lose?

A safe rate of weight loss is 1 to 2 pounds (0.45 to 0.9 kg) per week and is recommended for obese individuals. A slightly slower weight loss of 1/2 pound (0.23 kg) per week may be appropriate for those who are overweight. This rate helps promote fat loss while retaining muscle mass. When weight is lost more rapidly, the additional loss will be from fluid, muscle and liver glycogen, and muscle protein, rather than from fat. Weight lost at this slow rate is more likely to be permanent than if it is lost faster. Most people who lose large amounts of weight or lose weight rapidly eventually regain all that they have lost.

What Does It Take to Lose a Pound?

In order to decrease body fat, energy intake must be less than energy output. It is estimated that a pound of body fat provides 3,500 calories. Therefore, to lose a pound of fat, you must decrease energy intake by this amount, increase energy output by this amount, or use a combination of decreased intake and increased output to shift energy balance by 3,500 calories. To lose a pound in a week, you would need to shift energy balance by 500 calories per day (500 cal/day x 7 days in a week = 3,500 calories or 1 pound per week). This is the predicted average weight loss; however, the actual amount of weight lost per week may vary over time.

Is Weight Loss Safe for Everyone?

Weight loss diets are generally not recommended for children, pregnant women, or older adults. Children need a nutritionally adequate diet in order to continue their growth in height and their physiological development. Restricting calorie intake can interfere with growth. Therefore, it is generally recommended that young children who are overweight limit their calorie intake slightly and increase their exercise to stop weight gain. The goal is for them to continue to grow in height without gaining too much weight, so they will eventually have a BMI in the healthy range. A more extensive discussion of weight management in children is included in Chapter 9.

Weight loss is not recommended during pregnancy. Even women who are overweight at the start of pregnancy should gain at a slow, steady rate to accumulate about 15 to 25 pounds (7 to 11 kg) over the course of pregnancy. A weight loss program can be initiated after the baby is born and the mother has recovered. Slow weight loss is appropriate during lactation, but rapid weight loss can decrease milk production.

For older adults, the risks associated with excess body fat are lower than they are for younger adults.[33] However, the decision to treat obesity should not be based on age alone. Weight loss can enhance day-to-day functioning and improve cardiovascular disease risk factors at all ages. Older people tend to lose muscle and replace it with fat; therefore, weight-training activities are an important part of a weight loss program for the elderly.

WHAT IS A GOOD WEIGHT LOSS PLAN?

There are thousands of diets and programs available to promote weight loss. Some recommend specific foods, some provide lots of peer support, and some offer a detailed exercise plan. For some plans, you just need to buy a book and follow the diet plan, others have weekly meetings, and some guide you over the Internet. Which one will work best for you depends on your personal style—do you like working in groups or do you prefer to tackle challenges alone? It also depends on your lifestyle—do you travel frequently? Are you busy all day and only have time to yourself in the evening? Whichever type of program you choose, you will be most successful if you combine a reduced-calorie diet with an exercise regimen that increases expenditure and a program of behavior change that promotes weight management (Table 7.2). For people who have a BMI greater than 30 kg/m^2, drug therapy is often recommended, and for those with a BMI over 40 kg/m^2, weight loss surgery is an option.

Decreasing Intake

To lose weight, you need to eat fewer calories than you burn. But to lose weight safely, your diet must be low in calories while still providing all the nutrients your body needs. Drastic restrictions in food intake make it difficult to meet nutrient needs. The general recommendation for weight reduction is to reduce energy intake by 250 to 500 calories per day. Even without changing exercise patterns,

Table 7.2—What to Look for in a Weight Management Program

A healthy dietary pattern that can be followed for life

- Does the diet plan meet all your nutrient needs?

- Can the diet plan meet individual health needs? For example, can it be used by someone who has diabetes or high blood cholesterol?

- Does the program include an educational component to teach you how to make healthy food choices?

- Does the program take into consideration your eating habits and preferences?

- Is the diet plan flexible enough to be followed in different settings and on different occasions?

- Does the diet require you to purchase special foods or supplements?

Reasonable weight loss

- Does the program set realistic weight loss goals—a loss of 1/2 to 2 pounds per week?

Physical activity

- Does the program stress the need for you to increase physical activity?

Behavior change

- Does the program include some type of social support?

- Does the program promote changes in behavior that you can maintain over the long term?

Scientifically sound

- Is the program based on sound scientific principles?

- Are the personnel monitoring the weight management program health professionals?

Adapted from the American Heart Association's website. Available online at *http://www.amhrt.org/Health/Risk_Factors/Overweight/Fad_Diets/fadguide.html.*

this should produce a weight loss of 1/2 to 1 pound (0.23 to 0.45 kg) per week in most people—the rate of weight loss that promotes a loss of body fat, not lean body mass.

When reducing energy intake, choosing a nutrient-dense diet becomes very important. Foods must provide plenty of vitamins and minerals with few calories. For example, a salad with sliced chicken is a more nutrient-dense choice than a burger and fries. The diet should take into account the individual's risk for obesity-related diseases, such as cardiovascular disease, and follow the recommendations of the Dietary Guidelines. With energy intakes of fewer than 1,200 calories per day, a multivitamin and mineral supplement is recommended to ensure that nutrient needs are met. Medical super-vision is recommended if intake is 800 calories per day or less.

Increasing Activity

The other side of the energy balance equation is energy expenditure. Increasing energy expenditure through physical activity is an impor-tant component of any well-designed weight management program. Exercise increases the number of calories your body needs, so even if your intake is not reduced, fat stored in your body will be used for fuel. Exercise also promotes muscle development. This is important during weight loss because muscle is metabolically active tissue—it uses more calories to maintain itself than fat does. Increasing the amount of muscle you have helps to prevent the drop in BMR that occurs as body weight decreases. In addition to increasing energy expenditure, exercise improves overall fitness and relieves boredom and stress. Weight loss is better maintained when physical activity is included in the weight management program.[34] An increase in activity of just 100 calories a day will result in the loss of a pound in about a month.

Changing Behavior

Reducing energy intake and increasing exercise requires a change in behavior. In order to manage weight at a healthy level, this new behavior pattern must become part of your daily life for the long term. But changing behaviors is difficult. It requires identifying the old patterns that led to weight gain and replacing them with new ones to promote and maintain weight loss. This can be accomplished through a process called **behavior modification**, which is based on

---

FACT BOX 7.1

Two 1,500-calorie Choices

If you reduce the number of calories you consume, you will lose weight. It doesn't matter if the calories you take in come from a few high-calorie foods or many low-calorie choices. Each of the two diets in this chart provides 1,500 calories, but one has a lot more food than the other. Which diet would you rather eat?

	LOTS OF FOOD	A LITTLE FOOD
BREAKFAST	Cheerios®	Fried eggs
	Skim milk	Sausage
	Banana	Toast with butter
	Orange juice	
	Coffee	Coffee
LUNCH	Turkey sandwich with lettuce, tomato, and mustard	Hamburger on bun with lettuce, tomato, ketchup, mustard, and mayonnaise
	Apple	
	Skim milk	Soda
DINNER	Baked chicken breast	Fried chicken breast
	Baked potato with butter	
	Green salad with dressing	
	Brownie	
	Skim milk	

the theory that behaviors involve antecedents that lead to a behavior, the behavior itself, and the consequences of the behavior. These are referred to as the "ABCs" of behavior modification. For example, do you walk in the door after school or work and immediately go to the cookie jar and eat a handful of cookies? Afterward, do you regret that you ate more than you wanted? This behavior chain involves the antecedent—walking in the door hungry and opening the cookie jar; the behavior—eating the handful of cookies; and the consequence— feeling guilty because you ate more than you wanted. The key to modifying the behavior is to recognize the antecedent, so that the behavior and consequences can be changed. For example, plan a healthy snack ahead of time so when you walk in the door starving you won't go to the cookie jar. Instead, have some fruit salad or cut-up vegetables waiting for you. After eating the healthy snack, you will feel satisfied and pleased that you have added nutrient-dense foods and few calories to your day. Applying behavior modification techniques to change eating behaviors has been shown to improve

---

FACT BOX 7.2

How Can You Increase Energy Expenditure by 100 Calories a Day?

- Ride your bike for 20 minutes

- Spend 30 minutes bowling

- Walk for 30 minutes

- Spend 30 minutes cleaning your house

- Play tennis for 15 minutes

- Dance for 30 minutes

- Play basketball for 15 minutes

- Mow the lawn

long-term weight maintenance, as have other techniques, including stress management and stimulus control.

SUGGESTIONS FOR WEIGHT GAIN

As difficult as weight loss is for some people, weight gain can be equally elusive for underweight individuals. The first step toward weight gain is a visit to the doctor to rule out medical reasons for low body weight. This is particularly important when weight loss occurs unexpectedly. If the low body weight is due to low energy intake or high expenditure and not a medical problem, gradually increasing consumption of energy-dense foods is suggested. More frequent meals and high-calorie snacks such as peanut butter sandwiches or milkshakes between meals can help increase energy intake. Replacing low-calorie fluids like water and diet beverages with fruit juices and milk may also help. Strength-training exercise should be a component of any weight gain program. Keep in mind, however, that extra calories are needed to fuel the muscle-building activities.

These recommendations apply to individuals who are naturally thin and have trouble gaining weight on the recommended energy intake. This dietary approach will not result in weight gain in those who refuse to eat because of an eating disorder.

CONNECTIONS

Weight management involves developing healthy eating habits and maintaining active lives that promote the maintenance of a healthy weight. Weight management is important for everyone, even those who are currently at a healthy weight. To determine if someone should lose weight, his or her weight must be evaluated, along with his or her medical history, family history, and lifestyle factors. For those who would benefit from weight loss, an initial loss of 10% of current weight is recommended. More weight loss may be recommended if it is needed to further reduce health risks. Losing weight at a slow rate of about 1/2 to 2 pounds per week has been shown to promote the loss of fat while retaining muscle. Reducing intake and/or increasing activity by 3,500 calories will result in the loss of a pound (0.45 kg) of fat. A program that combines reduced intake with increased exercise and attention to behavioral changes to promote weight loss or maintenance has been shown to be the most effective way to manage weight. For those who need to gain weight, an increase in higher-calorie foods at meals and snacks combined with weight training can be used.

8

Diets and Other Weight Loss Fixes

Are you going on a diet? To most of us this means we are trying to reduce our energy intake to lose weight. But, if you "go on a diet," it implies that you will "go off the diet." Even if you lose weight, when you stop dieting and resume your previous eating pattern, you will most likely gain the weight back. This "on again, off again" pattern may allow you to look good for the prom, but it isn't what you need for weight management. To manage your weight at a healthy level, you need to establish a pattern of food intake and exercise that allows you to enjoy foods and activities you like without your weight climbing. If you are looking for a healthy weight loss program, it is important to find one that has a documented success rate and also meets your needs in terms of cost, convenience, and time commitment. Although many quick-fixes are tempting—what dieter wouldn't want to lose 10 pounds in just 2 days?—they are unlikely to promote long-term success at weight management (Table 8.1). For some people, even the best weight management program is not enough to help them lose weight and lower their

Table 8.1—Advantages and Disadvantages of Some Weight Loss Programs

PROGRAM	APPROACH	ADVANTAGES	DISADVANTAGES
Weight Watchers®	Low energy, social support	Safe, inexpensive, flexible	Requires group participation
Slim-Fast®	Low energy	Safe	Does not promote long-term behavior change
Optifast®	Low-calorie formula	Rapid weight loss	Expensive, dangerous if does not include medical supervision
Fit or Fat	Increased exercise	Safe, inexpensive	No social support
The Zone Diet	Low carbohydrate (40% of energy)	Inexpensive, flexible	Based on questionable principles, no social support
Eating Thin for Life	Moderation—written as weight loss success stories, recipes, and menu ideas	Inexpensive	No social support
South Beach Diet™	Initially low-carbohydrate, then limited carbohydrates are allowed	Safe, inexpensive, heart healthy	Initial weight loss is mostly water, no social support
Cabbage Soup Diet	Unlimited amounts of cabbage soup, fruit, coffee, and tea	Rapid weight loss	No social support, does not promote long-term behavior change, lack of variety
Sugar Busters®	Eliminates sugar; low-calorie—1,200 Cal a day	Inexpensive	No social support, based on unsound principles, insufficient carbohydrate
Volumetrics Weight Control Plan	Emphasizes foods high in water, fiber, and air to promote fullness with few calories	Safe, inexpensive	No social support or exercise component
Atkins Diet™	Very low-carbohydrate	Inexpensive, rapid initial weight loss	No social support, insufficient carbohydrate
Slim for Life	Calorie reduction with increased exercise	Safe, taught by a dietitian, inexpensive	Requires group participation

health risks. Prescription medications that help reduce food intake may be helpful in some individuals. In cases of morbid obesity, surgery is an option when conventional approaches fail.

WHAT IS A HEALTHY DIET?

Whether you are trying to lose weight, gain weight, or maintain your weight, the principles of choosing a healthy diet are the same. A healthy diet is one that provides the right number of calories to keep you losing, gaining, or maintaining your weight so it is in the desirable range. It is a diet that provides the proper balance of carbohydrate, protein, and fat choices; plenty of water; and sufficient but not excessive amounts of essential vitamins and minerals. It is a diet that minimizes your risk of developing chronic diseases such as heart disease, cancer, and osteoporosis. Generally, recommendations from the Food Guide Pyramid and the Dietary Guidelines suggest a diet that is rich in whole grains, fruits, and vegetables; high in fiber; moderate in fat and sodium; and low in saturated fat, cholesterol, *trans* fat, and added sugars. Choosing this diet doesn't mean giving up your favorite foods. But it does require considering variety and balance.

Choosing a variety of foods is important because, even within food groups, different foods provide different nutrients. For example, strawberries are a fruit that provides vitamin C but little vitamin A, whereas apricots provide a source of vitamin A, but less vitamin C. If you choose only strawberries, you will get plenty of vitamin C but may be lacking in vitamin A. Balancing your diet means choosing foods that complement each other. This requires considering the nutrient density of foods you choose. Foods low in nutrient density such as baked goods, snack foods, and sodas should be balanced with nutrient-dense choices such as salads, fresh fruit, and large vegetable servings. If this type of balance is maintained, a weight loss diet need not exclude favorite foods. An occasional bag of chips or ice cream cone won't destroy a weight loss diet if it is balanced with lower-calorie choices at other times. But when you are trying to lose weight, choosing more nutrient-dense foods, like salads and vegetables, will mean you can eat more food before you have reached your calorie limit. No single dietary component can make or break a diet. Rather, it is the overall pattern of dietary intake combined with lifestyle factors such as activity level that determines the relationship between your diet and your health.

PLANS THAT REDUCE CALORIES

Weight loss plans that are based on reducing calorie intake are the most common. Some recommend energy reduction without restricting the types of foods selected, some use exchange systems to plan calorie and nutrient intake, and others provide low-calorie portion-controlled packaged meals and formulas. A few even try unusual approaches such as jaw wiring to restrict intake to liquids that can be taken through a straw. The most successful plans are those that offer less dramatic dietary changes that can be maintained for a lifetime.

Just Eating Less

The most common type of diet recommends choosing low-calorie foods and reducing your intake of higher-calorie choices. These programs offer flexibility and variety, and can suit the food preferences of any consumer. Food choices can be varied, but to be successful, calorie intake needs to be monitored. The Weight Watchers point system fits into this category—it restricts intake to a specific number of points, which are based on the calorie, fat, and fiber content of each food, but does not specify the food sources of these points. The disadvantage is that these diets can be difficult to plan and may not meet nutrient needs unless they are based on some type of food selection guidelines.

The Food Guide Pyramid can provide the structure necessary to plan a balanced low-calorie diet. By using the low end of the range of suggested servings and making low-calorie choices, a healthy diet with as few as 1,200 calories can be planned. Food labels can be used to help select packaged foods that are appropriate for a low-calorie diet. Individuals consuming less than 1,200 calories per day may need a vitamin or mineral supplement to ensure that nutrient needs are met.

Following an Exchange Plan

Food exchanges are groups of foods that are similar in their energy and nutrient content so foods in the same group can be exchanged for one another. Diets that are based on exchanges recommend certain numbers of servings from specific food groups in order to provide a limited calorie intake but an adequate balance of nutrients. Some diet plans use the Exchange Lists established by the American Diabetes and American Dietetic associations. The benefit of this type of program is that the diet is more likely to meet nutrient needs than simply eating less, yet they still offer variety from meal to meal and from day to day. In addition, they teach meal-planning skills that are easy to apply away from home and can be used over the long term.

Pre-portioned Meal Plans

Many weight reduction diets provide pre-portioned packaged meals that are designed to replace some or all of the dieter's meals. Each meal contains a specific number of calories; these can be combined to provide the day's intake. Diets that rely on pre-packaged meals are easy to follow, but can be expensive and are not practical in the long term. Because all meals are provided,

---

FACT BOX 8.1

Calcium and Weight Loss

A recent review of popular diets showed that about half of the diet plans available today promote a diet that lacks calcium. This is bad for two reasons. First, adequate calcium intake is important for the prevention of the disease osteoporosis, which increases the risk of bone fractures in older adults. Second, a diet high in calcium may actually promote weight loss. Several recent studies have shown that as calcium intake increases, body weight decreases. This may be particularly true if the calcium comes from milk. Studies suggest that calcium from milk is twice as effective at reducing body fat as calcium from other sources.

Cross, Audrey. "Nutrition for the Working Woman." Available online at *http://www.fitcommerce.com*.

they do not teach the food selection skills needed to make a long-term lifestyle change.

Liquid Formula Diets

Rather than a pre-packaged meal, many diet plans rely on prepared liquid meals. Some of these regimens replace all meals with the liquid, while others recommend replacing only one or two meals per day. They can make reducing intake easy because they eliminate the problem of choosing low-calorie foods. Weight-loss regimens that rely exclusively on liquid formulas are not recommended without medical supervision. Most of these diets have high dropout rates and poor long-term weight-maintenance results.

Liquid weight loss formulas that are available over the counter are designed to be used in combination with food to provide a daily energy intake of about 800 to 1,200 calories. They can be effective if the foods eaten with them are low in calories. Although over-the-counter formulas are easy to use and relatively inexpensive, they do little to change eating habits for life.

SPECIAL FOODS OR FOOD COMBINATIONS

These types of diets focus on the supposed magical properties of specific foods or food combinations. For example, the grapefruit diet was based on the myth that grapefruit stimulates the breakdown of body fat. Diets that focus on food combinations and timing of intake are based on the faulty premise that foods should be eaten only in certain combinations and at certain times. They lead consumers to believe that if the rules are followed, body fat will melt away, but if foods are eaten in the wrong combination, they will not be digested properly, resulting in weight gain and disease. In reality, weight loss on such diets is due to the reduction in energy intake and not the magical properties of specific foods or combinations of foods. These types of diets may promote weight loss over the short term, but they cannot be consumed safely for long periods because the limited food can result in nutrient deficiencies. They also do not encourage exercise or promote the changes in eating behavior that are needed to affect body weight over the long term.

VERY-LOW-CALORIE DIETS

Someone who wants to lose weight very fast may be tempted to try a **very-low-calorie diet**. Very-low-calorie diets are defined as those containing fewer than 800 calories per day. They are a variation of the **protein-sparing modified fast**, which is a diet that provides little energy but has a high proportion of protein. Frequently, very-low-calorie diets are offered as a liquid formula that provides between 300 and 800 calories and 50 to 100 grams of protein per day and meets all other nutrient needs. The theory behind this is that the protein in the diet will be used to meet the body's protein needs and will, therefore, prevent excessive loss of body protein

Initial weight loss is rapid with very-low-calorie diets—3 to 5 pounds (1.4 to 2.3 kg) per week. This can provide a psychological boost and motivate the dieter to continue losing weight; however, in most cases, almost 75% of this initial weight loss is from water loss. Once the initial water loss ends, weight loss slows. The dieter's metabolic rate decreases to conserve energy and physical activity decreases because the dieter often does not have enough energy to continue his or her typical level of exercise.

Very-low-calorie diets are no more effective than other weight loss diets in the long term, and they carry more risks. When energy intake is as low as it is on these diets, body protein is broken down and potassium is excreted. A deficiency of potassium can cause the heart to beat irregularly and is potentially deadly. Other side effects include gallstones, fatigue, nausea, cold intolerance, light-headedness, nervousness, constipation or diarrhea, anemia, hair loss, dry skin, and menstrual irregularities. These diets are not recommended for people who are less than 30 to 40% above their healthy body weight, for pregnant or breast-feeding women, or for children, adolescents, or people with severe medical problems.[35] Since 1984, the FDA has required that all very-low-calorie diet formulas carry a warning that they can cause serious illness and should be used only under medical supervision.

LOW-FAT DIETS

Because fat is high in calories, consuming a low-fat diet typically reduces energy intake. Choosing low-fat foods such as grains, fruits, and vegetables can allow you to eat more food than you could with a high-fat diet providing the same number of calories. Differences in the way dietary fat and dietary carbohydrate are used by the body may also make low-fat diets more effective for weight loss. Dietary fat is stored efficiently as body fat, so consuming excess energy from fat leads to a greater accumulation of body fat than consuming excess energy as carbohydrate.[36]

Despite these advantages, low-fat diets don't always promote weight loss. A low-fat diet that includes large servings of rice, pasta, bread, and low-fat sweets can be high in calories. Even when a diet is low in fat, if you eat more calories than you burn, you will gain weight. The importance of total calorie consumption is illustrated by the fact that while the percent of fat calories in the typical American diet has decreased over the last few years, the number of people who are overweight continues to increase.

LOW-CARBOHYDRATE DIETS

The popularity of low-carbohydrate diets, such as the Atkins Diet, Sugar-Busters, and the South Beach Diet, has come and gone and returned again. In addition to promising weight loss, these diets claim to improve athletic performance and promote overall health. Some low-carbohydrate diets severely restrict carbohydrate intake by prohibiting foods such as breads, grains, and fruits, and limiting vegetable

---

FACT BOX 8.2

The First Low-Carbohydrate Diet

Before the Zone, Sugar-Busters, Protein Power, or even *Dr. Atkins' Diet Revolution*, there was the Banting diet. First published by William Banting in his 1864 book, *Letter on Corpulence*, this diet promoted a high-protein, high-fat, low-carbohydrate diet. Banting was an obese London undertaker whose health dramatically improved when he lost weight. He published the book at his own expense to make his diet available to everyone. The first 3 editions sold 63,000 copies in Great Britain alone. It was also translated and sold well in France, Germany, and the United States.

intake. They allow high-protein foods such as eggs, red meat, fish, and poultry in unlimited amounts. Other low-carbohydrate diets are less restrictive and limit carbohydrate intake to 40% of energy. Low-carbohydrate diets are based on the premise that excessive carbohydrate intake causes an increase in insulin, which promotes fat accumulation and stimulates hunger. Restricting carbohydrate consumption is hypothesized to reduce insulin, decrease hunger, and promote fat loss. Although it is true that blood insulin levels rise when carbohydrate is consumed, the regulation of body fat stores, hunger, and satiety depend on more than changes in insulin levels.

Despite the claims that carbohydrate-free foods can be eaten in unlimited amounts, weight loss occurs on these diets because intake is reduced. In some cases, weight is lost because the total amount of food allowed by the diet plan is limited; in other cases, it is lost

---

FACT BOX 8.3

Was Dr. Atkins Right?

The Atkins Diet has been around for a generation. This diet is high in fat and protein and severely limits carbohydrate intake. Nutritionists have criticized it for years. In 1973, the American Medical Association (AMA) called the diet dangerous and Dr. Robert Atkins had to testify before the U.S. Senate Select Committee on Nutrition. Despite its critics, the Atkins program continued to be a popular way to lose weight for over 30 years. Finally, in 2003, a study comparing the Atkins approach to a low-fat diet showed that after 6 months, obese patients had lost more weight using the Atkins Diet.[a] People on the Atkins Diet also had fewer risk factors for heart disease. Dr. Atkins, who fought for years to prove that he was right, died before the results were published. Will he be vindicated? A closer look at the results of this study show that although weight loss is greater after 6 months on the Atkins Diet, after a year, the difference disappeared and the weight loss was the same for both diets. There is currently a study under way to determine which diet works best for long-term weight management.

a Foster, G. D., H. R. Wyatt, J. O. Hill, B. G. McGuckin, C. Brill, B. S. Mohammed, P. O. Szapary, D. J. Rader, J. S. Edman, and S. Klein. "A randomized trial of a low-carbohydrate diet for obesity." *New England Journal of Medicine* 348 (2003): 2082–2090.

because boredom with the limited food choices causes a reduction in food intake. People following these diets experience an initial rapid weight loss, most of which is water. This occurs because, when carbohydrate intake is low, glycogen stores, along with the water they hold, are lost quickly. Ketones are produced because fat is not completely broken down in the absence of carbohydrate, and excretion of these ketones causes additional water loss. There is also some evidence that ketones in the blood suppress appetite, making it easier to reduce food intake. The risks associated with severe carbohydrate restriction are dehydration, potassium depletion, and ketosis. In addition, these diets are high in saturated fat, which promotes heart disease in the long term.

WEIGHT LOSS DRUGS

Most overweight people dream of a pill that will cause them to slim down without having to account for every morsel that goes in their mouth. An ideal drug to treat obesity would permit an individual to lose weight and maintain the loss, be safe when used for long periods of time, have no side effects, and not be addictive. Unfortunately, no such drug exists, but there are a variety of pharmaceutical products that have been developed for weight loss. Some are well studied and offer legitimate aids to weight loss; others are ineffective and even dangerous. Currently, drug treatment is only recommended for people whose health is seriously compromised by their excess body weight. Drug therapy should be considered for individuals with a BMI greater than 30 who do not have other obesity-related diseases and for those with a BMI greater than or equal to 27 who have other obesity-related diseases.[12]

Prescription Medications

Millions of Americans are taking medications prescribed to help with weight management. The most commonly used drug is phentermine. This medication decreases appetite by stimulating the hypothalamus and affecting the activity of certain neurotransmitters. Sibutramine (Meridia®) is another medication prescribed for weight loss. It also decreases food intake by affecting the activity of brain neurotransmitters that regulate food intake. Orlistat (Xenical®) acts via a different mechanism. It reduces energy intake by blocking fat-digesting enzymes in the intestine and hence reducing fat absorption. These drugs have shown promise at promoting weight loss in the short term, but the weight is regained when they are discontinued. There are also a number of drugs in various stages of development that may someday help reduce body weight by increasing energy expenditure, increasing the release of fat from adipose tissue, or decreasing fat synthesis.[37]

Over-the-Counter Medications

Only a limited number of substances are approved by the FDA for sale as nonprescription weight loss medications. These include fibers, benzocaine, and caffeine. Fibers such as methylcellulose and glucomannan are used in weight loss products because they absorb water to create a feeling of fullness; pills containing them claim to fill the stomach with indigestible bulk so that one feels full and eats less. The anesthetic benzocaine is included in weight loss products because it numbs the tongue, making eating a less pleasurable experience. Caffeine, which is a stimulant and a diuretic, is used in many

---

FACT BOX 8.4

Fen-phen Banned

Many attempts have been made to develop the perfect weight loss drug. In the 1990s, the drug combination fen-phen (fenfluramine and phentermine) successfully reduced appetite and appeared to make weight loss easier for many people. It seemed like a dream come true. In 1997, more than 18 million Americans, many of whom were only moderately overweight, were taking fen-phen when the bubble burst. The drug combination was linked to serious heart valve damage. As a result, fenfluramine and the related drug dexfenfluramine were withdrawn from the market. This series of events was a grim reminder to the weight-loss community that drugs carry risks and, in some cases, the drug risks outweigh the risks associated with excess body fat.

weight loss products because stimulants tend to blunt the appetite and diuretics cause the kidneys to increase fluid excretion, resulting in weight loss from water loss. These same effects can be derived from caffeine-containing beverages like coffee, tea, and some soft drinks. Most of these over-the-counter products are effective in the short term but do little to promote long-term weight loss.

Dietary Supplements

Common ingredients in weight loss dietary supplements include the amino acids arginine and ornithine, the mineral chromium, and a variety of herbs. Arginine and ornithine are hypothesized to burn fat during sleep because they stimulate the release of growth hormone. Although growth hormone promotes fat loss and muscle growth, research has not found any relationship between body weight and levels of growth hormone. Chromium is usually included as chromium picolinate. It is claimed to decrease body fat and increase the proportion of lean tissue, but human trials have not consistently demonstrated an effect of supplemental chromium picolinate on body composition or body weight.[38]

Weight loss supplements also often include herbal sources of compounds contained in prescription medications. Some of these are powerful drugs with dangerous side effects. Because they are sold as dietary supplements and not drugs, they are not strictly regulated; their safety and effectiveness may not have been carefully tested and doses may vary from tablet to tablet and brand to brand. It cannot be assumed that a product is safe simply because it is labeled "herbal" or "all natural." The FDA does not regulate dietary supplements for weight loss unless they claim to be a substitute for a drug or claim to perform a drug action or therapy.

Herbal ingredients that are used in weight loss products include bitter orange and green tea extract. Bitter orange contains a compound that is a central nervous system stimulant. It is similar to the banned diet herb ephedra, and, like ephedra, may cause side effects such as an increase in heart rate and blood pressure. Green tea extract contains chemicals that exaggerate the effects of bitter orange. It can cause jitters, insomnia, headaches, and gastrointestinal upset.

FACT BOX 8.5

The Dangers of Ephedra

Ephedra is an herbal extract that was used for years in dietary supplements that promised to promote weight loss or improve athletic performance. There is some evidence that it had small beneficial effects, particularly for weight loss. It can have serious side effects, however, including heart attack, stroke, and even death. Eventually, the FDA concluded that the dangers of ephedra outweighed its benefits and it became the first dietary supplement to be banned by the FDA.

The risks of ephedra came to light dramatically in February 2003 when 23-year-old baseball pitcher Steve Bechler died of heat stroke while taking an ephedra-containing supplement to lose weight. He collapsed during a training session in the hot, humid Florida weather and died the next day when his body temperature reached 108°F (42°C). An autopsy revealed ephedra, along with smaller amounts of two other stimulants—pseudoephedrine and caffeine—in his blood. Did ephedra cause Steve's death? No one can be sure he wouldn't have died even if he didn't take it. Steve was overweight and out of shape. He was not used to the hot weather. He was on a weight-loss diet and did not feel well or eat the night before he collapsed. He also had high blood pressure and some liver problems. These were certainly all factors, but ephedra constricts blood vessels in the skin and raises body temperature, perhaps by up to 2°F (-16.7°C). So, even though the official cause of death was heat stroke, ephedra may have played a role.

Bechler's case was not the first report of a serious problem associated with ephedra. A review of 16,000 reports of adverse effects revealed two deaths, four heart attacks, nine strokes, one seizure, and five psychiatric cases involving the supplement. Even before the FDA ordered ephedra-containing products off the shelves, it had been banned by minor league baseball, the National Football League, the National Collegiate Athletic Association, and the International Olympic Committee, but not by Major League Baseball.

Another type of herbal product marketed for weight loss is plant-derived laxatives. These are sold as teas or supplements and include senna, aloe, buckthorn, rhubarb root, cascara, and castor oil. Cascara, senna, and castor oil are approved by the FDA and regulated as drugs for use in nonprescription laxatives. These cause weight loss by inducing diarrhea, which causes water loss. They don't lead to fat loss, however, because they do not significantly reduce nutrient absorption. This is because they act in the colon, not in the small intestine, where most absorption occurs. Overuse of herbal laxatives can cause serious side effects, including nausea, diarrhea, vomiting, stomach cramps, chronic constipation, fainting, and severe electrolyte imbalances leading to cardiac arrhythmia and death.[39]

SURGERY

A more drastic method of weight management is surgery. This method has become increasingly popular over the last few years. Despite its increasing popularity, people should be aware that it is major surgery and having the procedure done does not solve the weight problem for you. Promoting and maintaining weight loss still requires significant lifestyle changes.

Who Is a Surgical Candidate?

Obesity surgery is recommended in cases where the risk of dying from obesity and its complications is great. It is appropriate only for individuals with a BMI greater than or equal to 40 kg/m^2 (extreme obesity) and those with a BMI between 35 and 40 kg/m^2 (obesity) who have other obesity-related conditions (see Table 7.1).[12] The success of weight loss surgery, as with other treatments, depends on the motivation and behavior of the patient. The appropriateness of surgery has to be evaluated on a case-by-case basis by considering the individual's potential risks and benefits.

Types of Surgery

The surgical approaches used to treat obesity include gastroplasty and gastric bypass (Figure 8.1). Gastroplasty involves stapling off the top part of the stomach to make it smaller. Gastric bypass

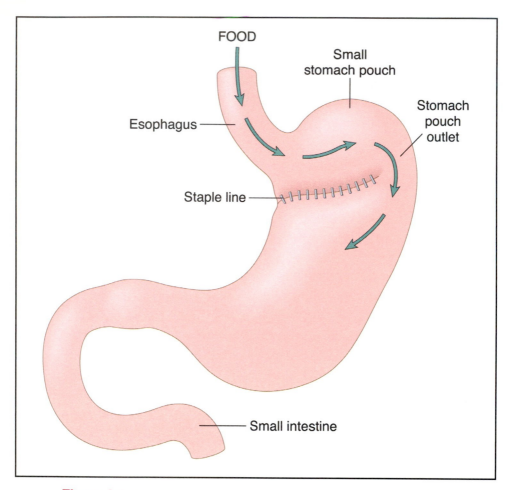

Figure 8.1 Gastroplasty, also known as stomach stapling, reduces food intake by decreasing the amount of food the stomach can hold. As seen here, a line of staples makes a small pouch in the stomach, preventing food from going into the rest of the stomach cavity.

involves bypassing part of the stomach by connecting the intestine to the upper portion of the stomach. In both cases, food intake is reduced because the now-smaller stomach becomes full after eating less food. Significant weight loss is usually achieved by 18 to 24 months after surgery. Some weight regain is common after two to five years. The success rate is lower with gastroplasty because the staples can be broken by consumption of large meals. Both of these procedures have short-term surgical risks and a long-term risk of nutrient deficiencies, particularly of vitamin B_{12}, folate, and iron.[40] To be successful, even such surgical procedures must be accompanied by behavior modification, diet programs, and exercise.

Another surgical approach, liposuction, is primarily a cosmetic procedure that will not significantly reduce overall body weight but may alter fat distribution. This procedure involves inserting a large hollow needle under the skin into a localized fat deposit and literally vacuuming out the fat. It is often advertised as a way to remove cellulite, which is fat that has a lumpy appearance because of the presence of connections to the tissue layers below.

CONNECTIONS

There are thousands of different weight loss diets and programs. To reduce body weight and maintain the loss, food intake patterns need to be changed for life. A diet that cannot be used for life will not maintain weight loss over the long term. When selecting a program, a person needs to choose one that will meet his or her personal preferences for food, activity, and social support. There are many ways to reduce calorie intake, including simply eating less; purchasing pre-portioned foods or liquid formulas that limit intake; reducing specific nutrients, such as carbohydrates or fat; and severely restricting total energy intake. When diet and exercise are not enough, there are drugs that may help reduce intake. Some are available by prescription only; others are over-the-counter medications or dietary supplements that may help reduce intake. There are also surgical methods of reducing food intake by making the stomach smaller. Surgery is generally recommended only when the risks associated with remaining obese are severe.

9

Weight Management in Children and Adolescents

The obesity crisis in the United States is not limited to the adult population; it is estimated that 15% of children and adolescents are overweight.[41] The incidence of obesity among adults has doubled since 1980, while the number of overweight adolescents has tripled. As with the adult population, this growing trend is likely to be the result of both an excessive intake of high-calorie foods and a lack of adequate physical activity.

The diagnosis and treatment of overweight and obesity in children and teens is more complex than in adults because they are still growing and developing. Whether an increase in weight is the precursor to a growth spurt or a concern for future health can be difficult to determine. If the child is overweight, weight loss planning can be challenging because of the importance of consuming a diet that supplies enough energy and the right amounts of essential nutrients to ensure normal growth and development. Consequently, different standards to define overweight and different approaches to managing weight have been developed for children and teens.

WHAT IS A HEALTHY WEIGHT FOR CHILDREN AND TEENS?

In adults, overweight and obesity are defined by whether BMI falls within the overweight or obese range. These BMI ranges are the same for both genders and all adult age groups. However, in individuals between the ages of 2 and 20, the definition of overweight is based on where BMI falls in relation to the BMIs of others of the same age and gender. A single standard cannot be applied to all age groups because the definition of a healthy weight varies with the stage of growth and development.

Consider Growth Patterns

From birth, healthy children follow standard patterns of growth. A child's growth can therefore be monitored by comparing his or her size to these standards. Growth charts that display typical growth patterns of infants, children, and adolescents in the United States have been developed by the Centers for Disease Control and Prevention (CDC). There are separate charts for infants from birth to 36 months of age and for children and adolescents from 2 to 20 years of age.[42] For infants from birth to 36 months of age, charts are available to monitor weight-for-age, length-for-age (measured lying down), head-circumference-for-age, and weight-for-length. For those over the age of 2 years, charts are available for weight-for-age, height-for-age, weight-for-height, and BMI for age (Appendix C).

By plotting a child's growth at various ages on a growth chart, his or her pattern of growth can be monitored and compared with that of other children of the same age. The resulting ranking, or percentile, indicates where the child falls in relation to population standards. There are variations in overall growth. For instance, Asian children are usually smaller than African-American and Caucasian children. Likewise, a child whose parents are 5 feet tall may not have the genetic potential to be 6 feet tall. However, most children and adolescents follow standard patterns of growth, so a child who is at the 50th percentile for length and 25th percentile for weight should continue to follow approximately these length and weight curves.

Watch for Abnormal Growth

The maximum size that an individual will attain is affected by genetic, environmental, and lifestyle factors. Whatever the genetic potential may be, adequate nutrition is essential for a child to reach that potential. Slight fluctuations in growth rate are normal, but a consistent pattern of not following the growth curve or a sudden change in growth pattern is cause for concern.

A child who is not consuming sufficient calories will first show a drop in weight, and if the deficiency continues, growth in height will slow or stop. A BMI of less than the 5th percentile is considered underweight. In contrast, a rapid increase in weight without an increase in height may be an indicator that a child is consuming more calories than he or she needs. This change in growth pattern should be evaluated to determine the causes. For children and teens, a BMI that is between the 85th and 95th percentiles on growth charts puts them at risk for becoming overweight. A BMI that is at the 95th percentile or above is defined as overweight. Obesity is not distinguished from overweight in children and teens (Figure 9.1).

WHAT ARE THE RISKS FOR OVERWEIGHT KIDS?

As with adult obesity, being overweight in childhood and adolescence increases the risks of chronic disease. Overweight children and teens may have high blood cholesterol, elevated blood pressure, and above normal blood glucose levels, which increases the probability that they will develop heart disease, hypertension, and diabetes. Overweight girls may have hormonal disturbances that increase their risk of certain cancers. In addition to its health impact, being overweight affects the psychosocial development of children.

Blood Cholesterol and Heart Disease

The recommended level for blood cholesterol in children ages 2 to 18 is less than 170 mg per 100 ml. In the United States today, many

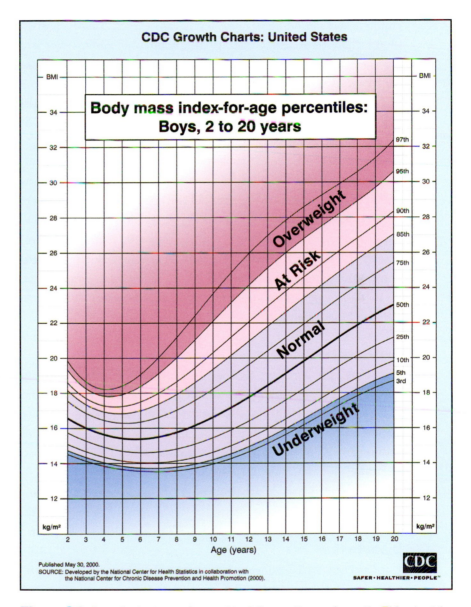

CDC Growth Charts: United States

Body mass index-for-age percentiles: Boys, 2 to 20 years

Published May 30, 2000.
SOURCE: Developed by the National Center for Health Statistics in collaboration with the National Center for Chronic Disease Prevention and Health Promotion (2000).

Figure 9.1 Growth charts can be used to follow patterns of growth. This chart for boys ages 2 to 20 shows the body mass index (BMI) values that are associated with underweight, normal weight, at risk of overweight, and overweight. A similar chart for girls 2 to 20 can be found in Appendix C.

(National Center for Health Statistics, National Center for Chronic Disease Prevention and Health Promotion, 2000) children have blood cholesterol levels that exceed this.[43] Elevated blood cholesterol levels during childhood and adolescence are associated with higher blood cholesterol and higher mortality rates from cardiovascular disease in adulthood.[44] The American Academy of Pediatrics recommends blood cholesterol monitoring for high-risk children and teenagers. This includes those with parents or grandparents who developed heart disease before age 55 and those whose parents have cholesterol levels over 240 mg per 100 ml.

Abnormal blood cholesterol levels are due to excess body fat as well as diet. Increased triceps skinfold thickness, which is a measure of body fat, is associated with increases in blood levels of LDL cholesterol ("bad" cholesterol) and decreases in HDL cholesterol ("good" cholesterol). The amount and type of dietary fat may also contribute to unhealthy cholesterol levels in children. As in adults, diets high in saturated fat, cholesterol, and *trans* fat can lead to elevated blood cholesterol levels in children.

Hypertension

High blood pressure may also be a concern early in life. Those who have blood pressure at the high end of normal as children are more likely to develop high blood pressure as adults.[45] Blood pressure can be affected by the amount of body fat, activity level, and sodium intake, as well as by the total pattern of dietary intake, so attention should be paid to these nutritional and lifestyle factors in children. This is particularly important if there is a family history of hypertension.

Diabetes

Until recently, type 2 diabetes was considered a disease that primarily affected adults over 40, but it is now on the rise among American youth.[9] The typical picture of type 2 diabetes in this population is a child age 10 to mid-puberty who is overweight and has a family history of the disease. Little is known about type 2 diabetes in children, but based on experience with adults, it is thought to be a progressive disease that increases in severity over time. The longer an individual has the disease, the greater the risk of complications that involve the circulatory system or nervous system and that can lead to blindness, kidney failure, heart disease, or amputations.

Preventive measures that may delay or prevent the onset of type 2 diabetes include weight management and increased physical activity for those at risk. The goal of treatment for diabetes is to keep blood glucose levels in the normal range by consuming a balanced diet that is moderate in energy and increasing physical activity.

Menstrual Problems and Early Menarche

Excess body fat causes hormonal abnormalities. In girls, this can affect the menstrual cycle; girls with higher body weights begin menstruation earlier than their leaner counterparts. Early **menarche** is a risk factor for breast cancer and is linked to cancers of the reproductive tract in women. It has also been proposed as a risk factor for psychiatric disorders common in adolescent girls, including depression, eating disorders, and substance abuse.[46]

Psychological and Social Consequences

Obese children and teens in the United States are less well accepted by their peers than normal-weight children and are frequently ridiculed and teased. They often have a poor self-image and low self-esteem. Children and adolescents who are overweight are typically stereotyped by their peers as having certain negative personality characteristics such as being lazy, sloppy, or stupid. The degree of this negative stereotyping increases with age. The fact that there are more overweight children and teens today than there were 40 years ago has not improved their social acceptance. A study done in 1961 had children rank drawings of children with various handicaps, indicating which ones they "liked best." The drawing of the obese child was ranked last among a drawing depicting a child with crutches, a child in a wheelchair, a child missing a hand, and a child with a facial disfigurement.[47] The study was recently repeated with similar results.[48]

Increased Risk for Eating Disorders

Children and teens who are overweight have a greater risk of developing an eating disorder than those who are of normal weight. Eating disorders are more prevalent in groups concerned with weight and body image, such as professional dancers and models.[49] It has been shown that eating disorders are more common in young females who diet to lose weight, whether or not their weight is in the normal range.

WEIGHT MANAGEMENT FOR CHILDREN AND TEENS

As with adult obesity, heredity, environment, and lifestyle all play a role in the development of childhood obesity. Obese parents are more likely to have offspring who become obese, not only because they pass on a genetic tendency to be overweight but because their children may learn poor eating and exercise habits. If sound nutrition and exercise habits are developed early and are followed throughout life, obesity can be avoided despite a genetic predisposition.

The goal of weight management in children and teens is to develop healthy eating and exercise patterns that will allow weight to be maintained in the normal range. For many children, this does not require weight loss. Slowing weight gain will be sufficient to allow the child to grow into his or her weight. For example, when the rate of weight gain is slowed but intake is sufficient to allow growth in height, a child at the 95th percentile for weight at age 7 can be at the 90th percentile by age 9 and at the 75th percentile by age 11. Children with a BMI greater than or equal to the 95th percentile and those with a BMI greater than or equal to the 85th percentile who have complications related to being overweight should undergo evaluation and possible treatment to reduce their body weight.[50]

Managing weight, whether this means losing weight, maintaining weight, or slowing weight gain, requires that energy intake and energy expenditure be modified. Changes in food intake and activity patterns should be gradual and should involve the entire family. If weight control at home is not effective, professional help may be needed.

Reducing Intake

In order to promote weight loss or prevent weight gain, a moderate calorie reduction may be necessary. Denying food, however, can promote overeating if the child feels he or she is being starved. To avoid this, a small reduction in calorie intake of only about 100 and 200 calories per day is recommended. Although slightly reduced in energy intake, this diet must provide adequate protein and micronutrients to allow growth. Nutrients that are of particular importance are vitamin A, vitamin C, vitamin E, calcium, iron, and zinc because they are likely to be deficient in the diets of children in the United States.[51] A diet that follows the recommendations of the Food Guide Pyramid will provide adequate vitamins and minerals (Figure 9.2). Children with particularly erratic eating habits may benefit from a multivitamin and mineral supplement that provides no more than 100% of the Daily Values. A healthy diet, rather than a restricted diet, should be stressed. Whole grains, fruits, and vegetables,

---

FACT BOX 9.1

10 Ways to Change Your Energy Balance by 100 Calories

1) Buy a smaller-sized bag of chips.

2) Skip dessert.

3) Bring your own lunch instead of buying lunch at school.

4) Instead of standing around at recess, walk around the track for 30 minutes.

5) Eat breakfast; you'll eat less later in the day.

6) Have an apple with lunch instead of a candy bar.

7) Spend 30 minutes riding your bike after school instead of watching television.

8) When you get home from school, have a glass of low-fat milk as a snack.

9) Take the bus—you'll get more exercise than if your mom drives you to school.

10) Have one scoop of ice cream rather than two.

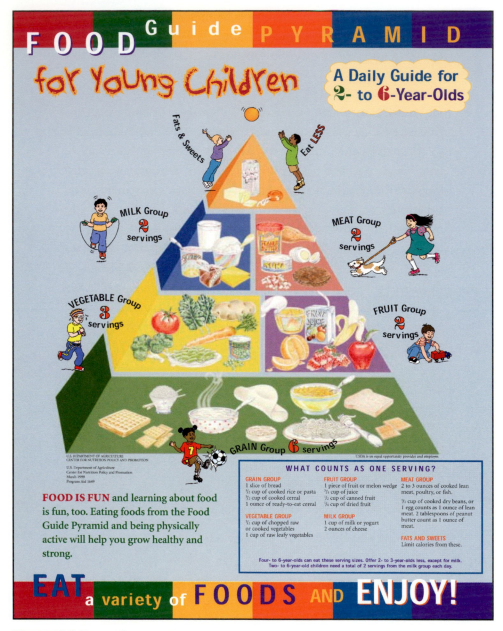

Figure 9.2 The nutrients and food portions young children need differ from those of adults. The Food Guide Pyramid for Young Children from the U.S. Department of Agriculture's Center for Nutrition Policy and Promotion can help plan healthy diets for 2- to 6-year-old children.

lean meats, and reduced-fat dairy products should be offered at meals and high-calorie, high-fat snacks should be limited. Following the serving recommendations and selection tips of the Food Guide Pyramid can help plan such a diet.

Increasing Activity

All healthy children should be physically active. Most are naturally active; extended periods of inactivity are not normal for healthy children. Promoting an increase in physical activity may be even more important than limiting intake when treating overweight children and adolescents. Although energy intake among American youth overall is not increasing, young people are getting heavier, suggesting that a major contributor to the increase in body weight is a lack of physical activity.[52] Some of this decrease in activity has come about because watching television, playing video games, and surfing the Internet have replaced neighborhood games of tag and soccer. Other sociocultural factors such as long days at school, living in single-family households, and unsafe outdoor environments have also contributed to inactive lifestyles.

FACT BOX 9.2

Sweetened Drinks Add Pounds

A recent study found that children who daily drank more than 12 ounces (0.35 liters) of sweetened beverages, such as soda and fruit drinks, gained a lot more weight than children who drank less than 6 ounces (0.18 liters) a day. The difference in weight was due to the fact that the children did not reduce how much food they ate at meals to make up for the calories they took in by drinking the sweetened drinks. The more sweetened drinks they drank, the greater their daily calorie intake and the greater their weight gain. Researchers also found that the more sweetened beverages the children consumed, the less milk they drank because, when offered a choice between sweetened drinks and milk, they chose the sweetened drink.

Source: Available online at *http://www.human.cornell.edu/faculty/facultybio.cfm?netid=dal4&facs=1.*

Overweight children and adolescents are less likely to be physically active than lean children. They often feel inadequate when participating in sports and teasing may further reduce their motivation to take part. They may be embarrassed by their bodies and shy away from taking part in group activities. A good way to get them moving is to encourage activities such as games, walks after dinner, bike rides, hikes, swimming, and volleyball that can be enjoyed by the whole family. This sends a positive message to "be more active" rather than a negative message of "do not eat so much." An exercise program is most effective if the activities are enjoyable. To make exercise a positive experience, increases in physical activity need to be gradual. Involvement of the whole family is key; parents who are active, play with their children, watch their children compete or play, or take children to physical activities or sports events have more active children.[53]

The National Association for Sports and Physical Education recommends that preadolescent children be physically active for at least an hour and up to several hours per day.[54] Children have short attention spans, so their activities should be intermittent. Periods of moderate to vigorous activity lasting 10 to 15 minutes or more each day should be interspersed with periods of rest and recovery. Children should be exposed to many different types of activities at varying levels of intensity.

Adolescents who are already active should be encouraged to remain active, and those who are inactive should be counseled as to how they can increase their activity level. Some enjoy organized team sports but these are not the only way to maintain an active lifestyle. Skating, skiing, cycling, swimming, power- or race-walking, tennis, aerobic dancing, kickboxing, Tae Bo®, rowing, racquetball, and handball are some other options. Adolescents should be involved in the decision-making process so they can select the activities they enjoy most. As with children, role models are important. Parents who encourage a teen to exercise should set the example by exercising themselves. Learning to enjoy exercise during childhood and adolescence will set the stage for an active lifestyle and weight management in adulthood.

Reducing TV Time

Television and computer games are part of American childhood today. Children spend more time watching television than they do in school.[55] As a result, it has become a lifestyle factor that influences children's nutrition and health. Through advertising, television has a strong influence on the foods young children select. A review of commercials broadcast during children's programming found that over 60% were for food products—primarily sweetened breakfast cereals; sweets such as candy, cookies, donuts, and other desserts; snacks; and beverages—that are high in sugar, fat, or salt.[56] Television also promotes snacking behavior.[56] Although snacks are an important part of a growing child's diet, many children snack on sweet and salty foods that are low in nutrient density while watching television.

Perhaps the most important nutritional influence of television is that it reduces activity. Hours spent watching television are hours when physical activity is at a minimum. One study showed that children who watch four or more hours of television per day have a

---

FACT BOX 9.3

How Much Does Activity Affect Energy Needs?

If you increase your overall level of physical activity, you need to eat more to maintain your weight. Using the EER equation shown below you can calculate that a sedentary 16-year-old girl who is 5 feet, 4 inches (1.6 meters) tall and weighs 127 pounds (58 kg) needs to eat only 1,770 calories a day to maintain her weight. If she adds an hour of moderate activity to her day, she will be in the active PA category and will need to increase her food intake to 2,420 calories per day to maintain her weight. If she joins the soccer team and gets 2 hours of vigorous exercise at practice every day, she will need to increase her intake to 2,940 calories or more per day. The formula below is for a 16-year-old female.

EER = 135.3 − (30.8 x Age in yrs) + PA [(10.0 x Weight in kg) + (934 x Height in m)] + 25

PA = sedentary 1.0, active 1.31, very active 1.56

greater amount of body fat and a greater BMI than those who watch fewer than two hours a day.[57]

DANGEROUS WEIGHT LOSS PRACTICES

Because children need energy and nutrients to continue their growth and development, severe approaches to weight loss can be dangerous. Sometimes weight goals are set based on peer pressure. Other times, they are set in order to meet weight guidelines or optimize performance in sports. Sports with weight categories such as wrestling may require an athlete to gain or lose weight to fit into a specific weight category. Weight loss is more common because competing at the high end of a weight class is believed to give a competitor an advantage over smaller opponents. Athletes may use dehydration to reduce weight rapidly. This is accomplished through such practices as vigorous exercise, fluid restriction, wearing vapor-impermeable

---

FACT BOX 9.4

Death of Three Young Wrestlers

In 1997, during a period of a little over than a month, three young wrestlers died while trying to "make weight." [a] They were exercising while wearing rubber suits to sweat off enough water to qualify for a lighter weight class. The deaths were caused by an increase in blood potassium concentration, which stops the heart. Muscle fibers that are damaged by heat release potassium. Normally, potassium levels in the blood are precisely regulated, but with dehydration, blood flow through the kidneys is reduced, so blood potassium levels increase. It is possible that some type of medication or supplement also played a role, but exercising in the heat is dangerous and, as a result of these three deaths, wrestling weight classes were altered to eliminate the lightest weight class, plastic sweat suits were banned, wrestling room temperatures could be no warmer than 75°F (24°C), weigh-ins were moved to one hour before competition, and mandatory weight loss rules were put in place to restrict the amount of weight that can be lost before a match.

a Information available online at *http://www.cin.org/archives/cinhealth/199901/0044.htm.*

suits, and using hot environments such as saunas and steam rooms. More extreme measures include vomiting and the use of diuretics and laxatives. These practices can be dangerous and even fatal. They may reduce performance and can adversely affect heart and kidney function, temperature regulation, and electrolyte balance. Athletes often think they can dehydrate for the weigh-in and then rehydrate in time for competition. However, the time between weigh-in and competition is not sufficient for fluid and electrolyte balance to return to normal in the muscles, or for the rehydration and replenishment of muscle and liver glycogen.[58]

CONNECTIONS

The number of overweight children in the United States is increasing. It is estimated that 15% of children and adolescents in the United States are currently overweight. In children and adolescents, body weight is assessed by using growth charts to compare a child's BMI with that of other children of the same age and sex. Healthy weight management can be difficult for children and teens because they must consume enough calories and nutrients to fulfill their growth potential. Too little energy can cause a decrease in growth. Too much energy can result in overweight. Overweight in children and teens increases the risk of chronic diseases such as heart disease, diabetes, high blood pressure, hormonal disturbances that can increase the risk of certain cancers, and difficulties in psychosocial development. The goal of weight management in children and teens is to develop healthy eating and exercise patterns that will allow weight to be maintained in the normal range for a lifetime. In some cases, rather than weight loss, the goal is to prevent weight gain and allow the child to grow into his or her weight. If calories are limited, the restriction should be mild. Activity should be increased and sedentary activities such as watching television and playing video games should be decreased.

Appendices

Appendix A

Acceptable Macronutrient Distribution Ranges (AMDR) for Healthy Diets as a Percent of Energy

Age	Carbohydrate	Added sugars	Total Fat	Linoleic acid	α-Linolenic acid	Protein
1-3 y	45-65	≤25	30-40	5-10	0.6-1.2	5-20
4-18 y	45-65	≤25	25-35	5-10	0.6-1.2	10-30
≥ 19 y	45-65	≤25	20-35	5-10	0.6-1.2	10-35

Source: Institute of Medicine, Food and Nutrition Board. "Dietary Reference Intakes for Energy, Carbohydrates, Fiber, Fat, Protein, and Amino Acids." Washington, D.C.: National Academies Press, 2002.

Dietary Reference Intakes: Recommended Intakes for Individuals: Carbohydrates, Fiber, Fat, Fatty Acids, and Protein

Life Stage Group	Carbohydrate (g/day)	Fiber (g/day)	Fat (g/day)	Linoleic acid (g/day)	α-Linolenic acid (g/day)	Protein (g/kg/day)	Protein (g/day)
Infants							
0-6 mo	60*	ND	31*	4.4*†	0.5*‡	1.52*	9.1*
7-12 mo	95*	ND	30*	4.6*†	0.5*‡	1.5	13.5
Children							
1-3 y	130	19*	ND	7*	0.7*	1.10	13
4-8 y	130	25*	ND	10*	0.9*	0.95	19
Males							
9-13 y	130	31*	ND	12*	1.2*	0.95	34
14-18 y	130	38*	ND	16*	1.6*	0.85	52
19-30 y	130	38*	ND	17*	1.6*	0.80	56
31-50 y	130	38*	ND	17*	1.6*	0.80	56
51-70 y	130	30*	ND	14*	1.6*	0.80	56
> 70 y	130	30*	ND	14*	1.6*	0.80	56
Females							
9-13 y	130	26*	ND	10*	1.0*	0.95	34
14-18 y	130	26*	ND	11*	1.1*	0.85	46
19-30 y	130	25*	ND	12*	1.1*	0.80	46
31-50 y	130	25*	ND	12*	1.1*	0.80	46
51-70 y	130	21*	ND	11*	1.1*	0.80	46
> 70 y	130	21*	ND	11*	1.1*	0.80	46
Pregnancy	175	28*	ND	13*	1.4*	1.1	RDA+25g
Lactation	210	29*	ND	13*	1.3*	1.1	RDA+25g

ND = not determined
* Values are AI (adequate intakes)
† Refers to all n-6 polyunsaturated fatty acids
‡ Refers to all n-3 polyunsaturated fatty acids

Source: Institute of Medicine, Food and Nutrition Board. "Dietary Reference Intakes for Energy, Carbohydrates, Fiber, Fat, Fatty Acids, and Protein." Washington, D.C.: National Academies Press, 2002.

Dietary Reference Intake Values for Energy: Estimated Energy Requirement (EER) Equations and Values for Active Individuals by Life Stage Group

Life Stage Group	EER prediction equation	EER for Active Physical Activity Level (kcal/day)[a]	
		Male	Female
0 – 3 months	EER = (89 x weight of infant in kg – 100) + 175	538	493 (2 mo)[c]
4 – 6 months	EER = (89 x weight of infant in kg – 100) + 56	606	543 (5 mo)[c]
7 – 12 months	EER = (89 x weight of infant in kg – 100) + 22	743	676 (9 mo)[c]
1 – 2 years	EER = (89 x weight of infant in kg – 100) + 20	1046	992 (2 y)[c]
3 – 8 years			
male	EER = 88.5 – (61.9 x Age in yrs) + PA[b][(26.7 x Weight in kg) + (903 x Height in m)] + 20	1742 (6 y)[c]	
female	EER = 135.3 – (30.8 x Age in yrs) + PA[b][(10.0 x Weight in kg) + (934 x Height in m)] + 20		1642 (6 y)[c]
9 – 13 years			
male	EER = 88.5 – (61.9 x Age in yrs) + PA[b] [(26.7 x Weight in kg) + (903 x Height in m)] + 25	2279 (11 y)[c]	
female	EER = 135.3 – (30.8 x Age in yrs) + PA[b] [(10.0 x Weight in kg) + (934 x Height in m)] + 25		2071 (11 y)[c]
14 – 18 years			
male	EER = 88.5 – (61.9 x Age in yrs) + PA[b] [(26.7 x Weight in kg) + (903 x Height in m)] + 25	3152 (16 y)[c]	
female	EER = 135.3 – (30.8 x Age in yrs) + PA[b] [(10.0 x Weight in kg) + (934 x Height in m)] + 25		2368 (16 y)[c]
19 and older			
males	EER = 662 – (9.53 x Age in yrs) + PA[b][(15.91 x Weight in kg) + (539.6 x Height in m)]	3067 (19 y)[c]	
females	EER = 354 – (6.91 x Age in yrs) + PA[b][(9.36 x Weight in kg) + (726 x Height in m)]		2403 (19 y)[c]
Pregnancy			
14 –18 years			
1st trimester	Adolescent EER + 0		2368 (16 y)[c]
2nd trimester	Adolescent EER + 340 kcal		2708 (16 y)[c]
3rd trimester	Adolescent EER + 452 kcal		2820 (16 y)[c]
19 – 50 years			
1st trimester	Adult EER + 0		2403 (19 y)[c]
2nd trimester	Adult EER + 340 kcal		2743 (19 y)[c]
3rd trimester	Adult EER + 452 kcal		2855 (19 y)[c]
Lactation			
14 –18 years			
1st 6 mo	Adolescent EER + 330 kcal		2698 (16 y)[c]
2nd 6 mo	Adolescent EER + 400 kcal		2768 (16 y)[c]
19 – 50 years			
1st 6 mo	Adult EER + 330 kcal		2733 (19 y)[c]
2nd 6 mo	Adult EER + 400 kcal		2803 (19 y)[c]

[a] The intake that meets the average energy expenditure of individuals at a reference height, weight, and age.
[b] See table entitled "PA Values" to determine the PA value for various ages, genders, and activity levels.
[c] Value is calculated for an individual at the age in parentheses.

PA Values used to calculate EER

Physical Activity Level (PA)	Sedentary	Low active	Active	Very active
3 to 18 years				
Boys	1.00	1.13	1.26	1.42
Girls	1.00	1.16	1.31	1.56
≥ 19 years				
Men	1.00	1.11	1.25	1.48
Women	1.00	1.12	1.27	1.45

Source: Institute of Medicine, Food and Nutrition Board. "Dietary Reference Intakes for Energy, Carbohydrates, Fiber, Fat, Protein, and Amino Acids." Washington, D.C.: National Academies Press, 2002.

Appendix A

Dietary Reference Intakes: Recommended Intakes for Individuals: Vitamins

Life Stage Group	Vitamin A (µg/day)[a]	Vitamin C (mg/day)	Vitamin D (µg/day)[b,c]	Vitamin E (mg/day)[d]	Vitamin K (µg/day)	Thiamin (mg/day)	Riboflavin (mg/day)	Niacin (mg/day)[e]	Vitamin B6 (mg/day)	Folate (µg/day)[f]	Vitamin B12 (µg/day)	Pantothenic Acid (mg/day)	Biotin (µg/day)	Choline[g] (mg/day)
Infants														
0-6 mo	400*	40*	5*	4*	2.0*	0.2*	0.3*	2*	0.1*	65*	0.4*	1.7*	5*	125*
7-12 mo	500*	50*	5*	5*	2.5*	0.3*	0.4*	4*	0.3*	80*	0.5*	1.8*	6*	150*
Children														
1-3 y	**300**	**15**	5*	**6**	30*	**0.5**	**0.5**	**6**	**0.5**	**150**	**0.9**	2*	8*	200*
4-8 y	**400**	**25**	5*	**7**	55*	**0.6**	**0.6**	**8**	**0.5**	**200**	**1.2**	3*	12*	250*
Males														
9-13 y	**600**	**45**	5*	**11**	60*	**0.9**	**0.9**	**12**	**1.0**	**300**	**1.8**	4*	20*	315*
14-18 y	**900**	**75**	5*	**15**	75*	**1.2**	**1.3**	**16**	**1.3**	**400**	**2.4**	5*	25*	550*
19-30 y	**900**	**90**	5*	**15**	120*	**1.2**	**1.3**	**16**	**1.3**	**400**	**2.4**	5*	30*	550*
31-50 y	**900**	**90**	5*	**15**	120*	**1.2**	**1.3**	**16**	**1.3**	**400**	**2.4**	5*	30*	550*
51-70 y	**900**	**90**	10*	**15**	120*	**1.2**	**1.3**	**16**	**1.7**	**400**	**2.4**[h]	5*	30*	550*
> 70 y	**900**	**90**	15*	**15**	120*	**1.2**	**1.3**	**16**	**1.7**	**400**	**2.4**[h]	5*	30*	550*
Females														
9-13 y	**600**	**45**	5*	**11**	60*	**0.9**	**0.9**	**12**	**1.0**	**300**	**1.8**	4*	20*	375*
14-18 y	**700**	**65**	5*	**15**	75*	**1.0**	**1.0**	**14**	**1.2**	**400**[i]	**2.4**	5*	25*	400*
19-30 y	**700**	**75**	5*	**15**	90*	**1.1**	**1.1**	**14**	**1.3**	**400**[i]	**2.4**	5*	30*	425*
31-50 y	**700**	**75**	5*	**15**	90*	**1.1**	**1.1**	**14**	**1.3**	**400**[i]	**2.4**	5*	30*	425*
51-70 y	**700**	**75**	10*	**15**	90*	**1.1**	**1.1**	**14**	**1.5**	**400**	**2.4**[h]	5*	30*	425*
> 70 y	**700**	**75**	15*	**15**	90*	**1.1**	**1.1**	**14**	**1.5**	**400**	**2.4**[h]	5*	30*	425*
Pregnancy														
≤ 18 y	**750**	**80**	5*	**15**	75*	**1.4**	**1.4**	**18**	**1.9**	**600**[j]	**2.6**	6*	30*	450*
14-18 y	**770**	**85**	5*	**15**	90*	**1.4**	**1.4**	**18**	**1.9**	**600**[j]	**2.6**	6*	30*	450*
19-30 y	**770**	**85**	5*	**15**	90*	**1.4**	**1.4**	**18**	**1.9**	**600**[j]	**2.6**	6*	30*	450*
Lactation														
≤ 18 y	**1200**	**115**	5*	**19**	75*	**1.4**	**1.6**	**17**	**2.0**	**500**	**2.8**	7*	35*	550*
14-18 y	**1300**	**120**	5*	**19**	90*	**1.4**	**1.6**	**17**	**2.0**	**500**	**2.8**	7*	35*	550*
19-30 y	**1300**	**120**	5*	**19**	90*	**1.4**	**1.6**	**17**	**2.0**	**500**	**2.8**	7*	35*	550*

NOTE: This table (taken from the DRI reports, see www.nap.edu) presents Recommended Dietary Allowances (RDAs) in **bold** type and Adequate Intakes (AIs) in ordinary type followed by an asterisk (*). RDAs and AIs may both be used as goals for individual intakes. RDAs are set up to meet the needs of almost all (97–98%) individuals in a group. For healthy breastfed infants, the AI is the mean intake. The AI for all other life stage and gender groups is believed to cover needs of all individuals in the group, but lack of data or uncertainty in the data prevent being able to specify with confidence the percentage of individuals covered by this intake.

[a]As retinol activity equivalents (RAEs). 1 RAE = 1 µg retinol, 12 µg β-carotene, 24 µg β-carotene, or 24 µg β-cryptoxanthin in foods. To calculate RAEs from REs of provitamin A carotenoids in foods, divide RE by 2. For preformed vitamin A in foods or supplements and for provitamin A carotenoids in supplements, 1 RE = 1 RAE.

[b]Cholecalciferol. 1 µg cholecalciferol = 40 IU vitamin D.

[c]In the absence of exposure to adequate sunlight.

[d]As α-tocopherol, which includes RRR-α-tocopherol, the only form of α-tocopherol that occurs naturally in foods, and the 2R-stereoisomeric forms of α-tocopherol (RRR-, RSR-, RRS-, and RSS-α-tocopherol). Does not include the 2S-stereoisomeric forms of α-tocopherol (SRR-, SSR-, SRS-, and SSS- α -tocopherol), also found in food and supplements.

[e]As niacin equivalents (NEs), 1mg niacin = 60 mg tryptophan; 0-6 months = preformed niacin (not NE).

[f]As dietary folate equivalents (DFEs). 1 DFE = 1 µg food folate = 0.6 µg folic acid from fortified food or as a supplement consumed with food = 0.5 µg of a supplement taken on an empty stomach.

[g]Although AIs have been set for choline, there are few data to assess whether a dietary supplement of choline is needed at all stages of the life cycle, and it may be that the choline requirement can be met by endogenous synthesis at some of these stages.

[h]Because 10-30% of older people may malabsorb food-bound B12, it is advisable for those older than 50 years to meet their RFD mainly by consuming foods fortified with B12 or containing B12.

[i]In view of evidence linking folate intake with neural tube defects in the fetus, it is recommended that all women capable of becoming pregnant consume 400 µg from supplements or fortified foods in addition to intake of food folate from a varied diet.

[j]It is assumed that women will consume 400 µg from supplements or fortified foods until their pregnancy is confirmed and they enter prenatal care, which ordinarily occurs after the end of the periconceptional period – the critical time for neural tube formation.

Source: Trumbo, P., A. Yates, S. Schlicker. M. Poos. "Dietary Reference Intakes: Vitamin A, Vitamin K, Arsenic, Boron, Chromium, Copper, Iodine, Iron, Manganese, Molybdenum, Nickel, Silicon, Vanadium, and Zinc." _Journal of the American Dietetic Association_ 101, no. 3 (2001) 294-301.

Dietary Reference Intakes: Recommended Intakes for Individuals: Minerals

Life Stage Group	Calcium (mg/day)	Chromium (µg/day)	Copper (µg/day)	Fluoride (mg/day)	Iodine (µg/day)	Iron (mg/day)	Magnesium (mg/day)	Manganese (mg/day)	Molybdenum (µg/day)	Phosphorus (mg/day)	Selenium (µg/day)	Zinc (mg/day)
Infants												
0-6 mo	210*	0.2*	200*	0.01*	110*	0.27*	30*	0.003*	2*	100*	15*	2*
7-12 mo	270*	5.5*	220*	0.5*	130*	11	75*	0.6*	3*	275*	20*	3
Children												
1-3 y	500*	11*	340	0.7*	90	7	80	1.2*	17	460	20	3
4-8 y	800*	15*	440	1*	90	10	130	1.5*	22	500	30	5
Males												
9-13 y	1,300*	25*	700	2*	120	8	240	1.9*	34	1,250	40	8
14-18 y	1,300*	35*	890	3*	150	11	410	2.2*	43	1,250	55	11
19-30 y	1,000*	35*	900	4*	150	8	400	2.3*	45	700	55	11
31-50 y	1,000*	35*	900	4*	150	8	420	2.3*	45	700	55	11
51-70 y	1,200*	30*	900	4*	150	8	420	2.3*	45	700	55	11
>70 y	1,200*	30*	900	4*	150	8	420	2.3*	45	700	55	11
Females												
9-13 y	1,300*	21*	700	2*	120	8	240	1.6*	34	1,250	40	8
14-18 y	1,300*	24*	890	3*	150	15	360	1.6*	43	1,250	55	9
19-30 y	1,000*	25*	900	3*	150	18	310	1.8*	45	700	55	8
31-50 y	1,000*	25*	900	3*	150	18	320	1.8*	45	700	55	8
51-70 y	1,200*	20*	900	3*	150	8	320	1.8*	45	700	55	8
>70 y	1,200*	20*	900	3*	150	8	320	1.8*	45	700	55	8
Pregnancy												
≤18 y	1,300*	29*	1,000	3*	220	27	400	2.0*	50	1,250	60	13
14-18 y	1,000*	30*	1,000	3*	220	27	350	2.0*	50	700	60	11
19-30 y	1,000*	30*	1,000	3*	220	27	360	2.0*	50	700	60	11
Lactation												
≤18 y	1,300*	44*	1,300	3*	290	10	360	2.6*	50	1,250	70	14
14-18 y	1,300*	45*	1,300	3*	290	9	310	2.6*	50	700	70	12
19-30 y	1,300*	45*	1,300	3*	290	9	320	2.6*	50	700	70	12

NOTE: This table (taken from the DRI reports, see www.nap.edu) presents Recommended Dietary Allowances (RDAs) in **bold** type and Adequate Intakes (AIs) in ordinary type followed by an asterisk (*). RDAs and AIs may both be used as goals for individual intakes. RDAs are set up to meet the needs of almost all (97-98%) individuals in a group. For healthy breastfed infants, the AI is the mean intake. The AI for all other life stage and gender groups is believed to cover needs of all individuals in the group, but lack of data or uncertainty in the data prevents being able to specify with confidence the percentage of individuals covered by this intake.

Dietary Reference Intakes (DRIs): Tolerable Upper Intake Levels (UL[a]): Vitamins

Life Stage Group	Vitamin A (µg/day)[b]	Vitamin C (mg/day)	Vitamin D (µg/day)	Vitamin E (mg/day)[c,d]	Vitamin K	Thiamin	Riboflavin	Niacin (mg/day)[d]	Vitamin B₆ (mg/day)	Folate (µg/day)[d]	Vitamin B₁₂	Pantothenic Acid	Biotin	Choline (mg/day)	Carotenoids[e]
Infants															
0-6 mo	600	ND[f]	25	ND[f]	ND	ND	ND	ND	ND	ND	ND	ND	ND	ND	ND
7-12 mo	600	ND	25	ND	ND	ND	ND	ND	ND	ND	ND	ND	ND	ND	ND
Children															
1-3 y	600	400	50	200	ND	ND	ND	10	30	300	ND	ND	ND	1.0	ND
4-8 y	900	650	50	300	ND	ND	ND	15	40	400	ND	ND	ND	1.0	ND
Males, Females															
9-13 y	1,700	1,200	50	600	ND	ND	ND	20	60	600	ND	ND	ND	2.0	ND
14-18 y	2,800	1,800	50	800	ND	ND	ND	30	80	800	ND	ND	ND	3.0	ND
19-70 y	3,000	2,000	50	1,000	ND	ND	ND	35	100	1,000	ND	ND	ND	3.5	ND
>70 y	3,000	2,000	50	1,000	ND	ND	ND	35	100	1,000	ND	ND	ND	3.5	ND
Pregnancy															
≤18 y	2,800	1,800	50	800	ND	ND	ND	30	80	800	ND	ND	ND	3.0	ND
19-50 y	3,000	2,000	50	1,000	ND	ND	ND	35	100	1,000	ND	ND	ND	3.5	ND
Lactation															
≤18 y	2,800	1,800	50	800	ND	ND	ND	30	80	800	ND	ND	ND	3.0	ND
19-50 y	3,000	2,000	50	1,000	ND	ND	ND	35	100	1,000	ND	ND	ND	3.5	ND

[a]UL = The maximum level of daily nutrient intake that is likely to pose no risk of adverse effects. Unless otherwise specified, the UL represents total intake from food, water, and supplements. Due to lack of suitable data, ULs could not be established for vitamin K, thiamin, riboflavin, vitamin B₁₂, pantothenic acid, biotin, or carotenoids. In the absence of ULs, extra caution may be warranted in consuming levels above recommended intakes.

[b]As preformed vitamin A only.

[c]As α-tocopherol; applies to any for of supplemental α-tocopherol.

[d]The ULs for vitamin E, niacin, and folate apply to synthetic forms obtained from supplements, fortified foods, or a combination of the two.

[e]β-Carotene supplements are advised only to serve as a provitamin A source for individuals at risk of vitamin A deficiency.

[f]ND=Not determinable due to lack of data of adverse effects in this age group and concern with regard to lack of ability to handle excess amounts. Source of intakes should be from food only to prevent high levels of intake.

Dietary Reference Intakes (DRIs): Tolerable Upper Intake Levels (UL[a]): Minerals

Life Stage Group	Arsenic[b]	Boron (mg/day)	Calcium (g/day)	Chromium	Copper (μg/day)	Fluoride (mg/day)	Iodine (μg/day)	Iron (mg/day)	Magnesium (mg/day)[c]	Manganese (mg/day)	Molybdenum (μg/day)	Nickel (mg/day)	Phosphorus (g/day)	Selenium (μg/day)	Silicon[d]	Vanadium (mg/day)[e]	Zinc (mg/day)
Infants																	
0-6 mo	ND[f]	ND	ND	ND	ND	0.7	ND	40	ND	ND	ND	ND	ND	45	ND	ND	4
7-12 mo	ND	ND	ND	ND	ND	0.9	ND	40	ND	ND	ND	ND	ND	60	ND	ND	5
Children																	
1-3 y	ND	3	2.5	ND	1,000	1.3	200	40	65	2	300	0.2	3	90	ND	ND	7
4-8 y	ND	6	2.5	ND	3,000	2.2	300	40	110	3	600	0.3	3	150	ND	ND	12
Males, Females																	
9-13 y	ND	11	2.5	ND	5,000	10	600	40	350	6	1,100	0.6	4	280	ND	ND	23
14-18 y	ND	17	2.5	ND	8,000	10	900	45	350	9	1,700	1.0	4	400	ND	ND	34
19-70 y	ND	20	2.5	ND	10,000	10	1,100	45	350	11	2,000	1.0	4	400	ND	1.8	40
>70 y	ND	20	2.5	ND	10,000	10	1,100	45	350	11	2,000	1.0	3	400	ND	1.8	40
Pregnancy																	
≤18 y	ND	17	2.5	ND	8,000	10	900	45	350	9	1,700	1.0	3.5	400	ND	ND	34
19-50 y	ND	20	2.5	ND	10,000	10	1,100	45	350	11	2,000	1.0	3.5	400	ND	ND	40
Lactation																	
≤18 y	ND	17	2.5	ND	8,000	10	900	45	350	9	1,700	1.0	4	400	ND	ND	34
19-50 y	ND	20	2.5	ND	10,000	10	1,100	45	350	11	2,000	1.0	4	400	ND	ND	40

[a]UL= the maximum level of daily nutrient intake that is likely to pose no risk of adverse effects. Unless otherwise specified, the UL represents total intake from food, water, and supplements. Due to lack of suitable data, ULs could not be established for arsenic, chromium, and silicon. In the absence of ULs, extra caution may be warranted in consuming levels above recommended intakes.

[b]Although the UL was not determined for arsenic, there is no justification for adding arsenic to food or supplements.

[c]The ULs for magnesium represent intake from a pharmacological agent only and do not include intake from food and water.

[d]Although silicon has not been shown to cause adverse effects in humans, there is no justification for adding silicon to supplements.

[e]Although vanadium in food has not been shown to cause adverse effects in humans, there is no justification for adding vanadium to food and vanadium supplements should be used with caution. The UL is based on adverse effects in laboratory animals and this data could be used to set a UL for adults but not children and adolescents.

[f]ND=Not determinable due to lack of data of adverse effects in this age group and concern with regard to lack of ability to handle excess amounts. Source of intake should be from food only to prevent high levels of intake.

Appendix A

Dietary Reference Intakes: Recommended Intakes and Tolerable Upper Intake Levels (UL): Water, Potassium, Sodium, and Chloride

Life Stage Group	Water [a] (liters)	Potassium [a,b] (mg)	Sodium (mg)		Chloride (mg)	
			Recommended Intake	UL	Recommended Intake	UL
Infants						
0–6 mo	0.7	0.4	0.12	-	0.18	-
7–12 mo	0.8	0.7	0.37	-	0.58	-
Children						
1–3 y	1.3	3.0	1.0	1.5	1.5	2.3
4–8 y	1.7	3.8	1.2	1.9	1.9	2.9
Males						
9–13 y	2.4	4.5	1.5	2.2	2.3	3.4
14–18 y	3.3	4.7	1.5	2.3	2.3	3.6
19–30 y	3.7	4.7	1.5	2.3	2.3	3.6
31–50 y	3.7	4.7	1.5	2.3	2.3	3.6
51–70 y	3.7	4.7	1.3	2.3	2.0	3.6
>70 y	3.7	4.7	1.2	2.3	1.8	3.6
Females						
9–13 y	2.1	4.5	1.5	2.2	2.3	3.4
14–18 y	2.3	4.7	1.5	2.3	2.3	3.6
19–30 y	2.7	4.7	1.5	2.3	2.3	3.6
31–50 y	2.7	4.7	1.5	2.3	2.3	3.6
51–70 y	2.7	4.7	1.3	2.3	2.0	3.6
>70 y	2.7	4.7	1.2	2.3	1.8	3.6

[a] No UL has been established for water or potassium.

[b] The recommended intake is the same for all groups over 14 years except lactating women, which is 5.1 mg.

Metropolitan Life Insurance Weight for Height Tables

FRAME SIZE	SMALL	MEDIUM	LARGE
HEIGHT MEN*	WEIGHT (in pounds)		
5'2"	128–134	131–141	138–150
5'3"	130–136	133–143	140–153
5'4"	132–138	135–145	142–156
5'5"	134–140	137–148	144–160
5'6"	136–142	139–151	146–164
5'7"	138–145	142–154	149–168
5'8"	140–148	145–157	152–172
5'9"	142–151	148–160	155–176
5'10"	144–154	151–163	158–180
5'11"	146–157	154–166	161–184
6'0"	149–160	157–170	164–188
6'1"	152–164	160–174	168–192
6'2"	155–168	164–178	172–197
6'3"	158–172	167–182	176–202
6'4"	162–176	171–187	181–207
HEIGHT WOMEN†			
4'10"	102–111	109–121	118–131
4'11"	103–113	111–123	120–134
5'0"	104–115	113–126	122–137
5'1"	106–118	115–129	125–140
5'2"	108–121	118–132	128–143
5'3"	111–124	121–135	131–147
5'4"	114–127	124–138	134–151
5'5"	117–130	127–141	137–155
5'6"	120–133	130–144	140–159
5'7"	123–136	133–147	143–163
5'8"	126–139	136–150	146–167
5'9"	129–142	139–153	149–170
5'10"	132–145	142–156	152–173
5'11"	135–148	145–159	155–176
6'0"	138–151	148–162	158–179

* Weights at ages 25 to 59 based on lowest mortality.
  Weights in pounds according to frame (in indoor clothing weighing 5 lbs, shoes with 1 inch heels).

† Weights at ages 25 to 59 based on lowest mortality.
  Weights in pounds according to frame (in indoor clothing weighing 3 lbs, shoes with 1 inch heels).

Courtesy of Metropolitan Life Insurance Company

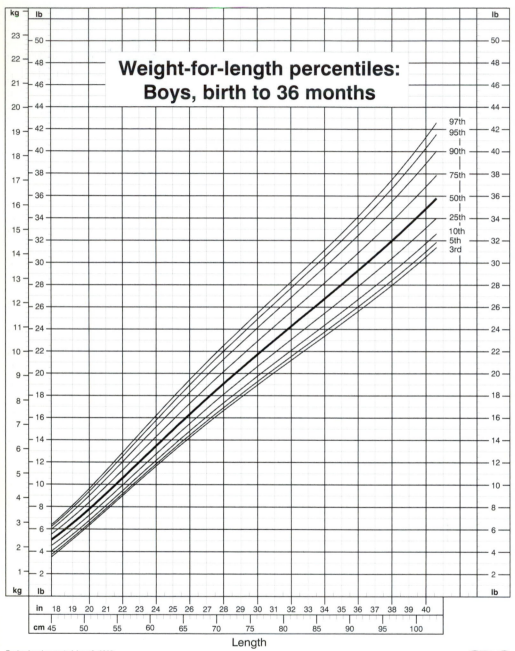

Weight-for-length percentiles: Boys, birth to 36 months

Length

Revised and corrected June 8, 2000.

SOURCE: Developed by the National Center for Health Statistics in collaboration with
the National Center for Chronic Disease Prevention and Health Promotion (2000).

CDC
CENTERS FOR DISEASE CONTROL
AND PREVENTION

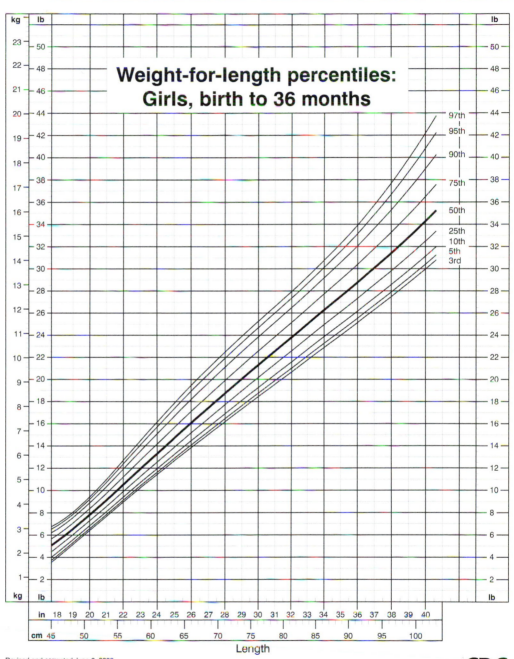

Weight-for-length percentiles: Girls, birth to 36 months

Revised and corrected June 8, 2000.

SOURCE: Developed by the National Center for Health Statistics in collaboration with the National Center for Chronic Disease Prevention and Health Promotion (2000).

CDC
CENTERS FOR DISEASE CONTROL
AND PREVENTION

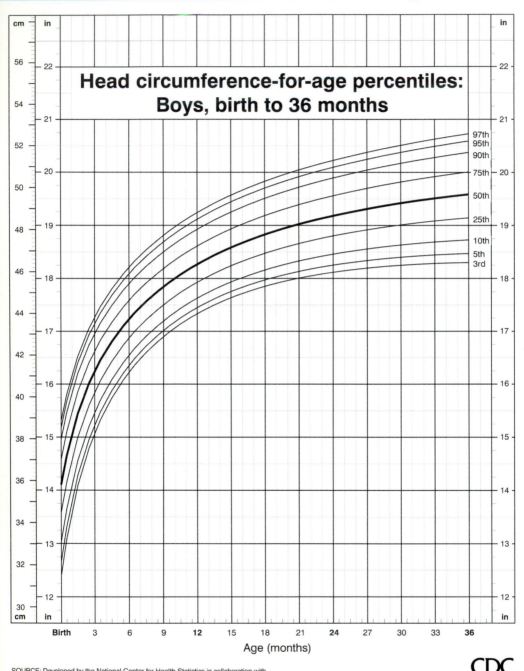

Head circumference-for-age percentiles: Boys, birth to 36 months

Age (months)

SOURCE: Developed by the National Center for Health Statistics in collaboration with the National Center for Chronic Disease Prevention and Health Promotion (2000).

CDC
CENTERS FOR DISEASE CONTROL AND PREVENTION

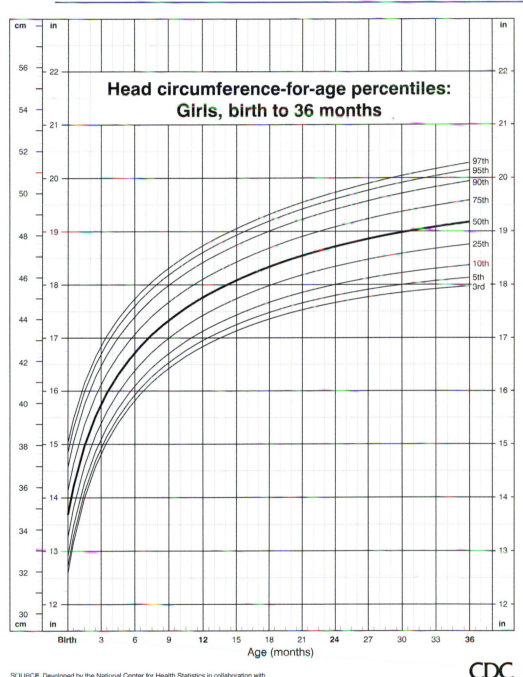

Head circumference-for-age percentiles:
Girls, birth to 36 months

97th
95th
90th
75th
50th
25th
10th
5th
3rd

Age (months)

Birth 3 6 9 12 15 18 21 24 27 30 33 36

SOURCE. Developed by the National Center for Health Statistics in collaboration with
the National Center for Chronic Disease Prevention and Health Promotion (2000).

CDC
CENTERS FOR DISEASE CONTROL
AND PREVENTION

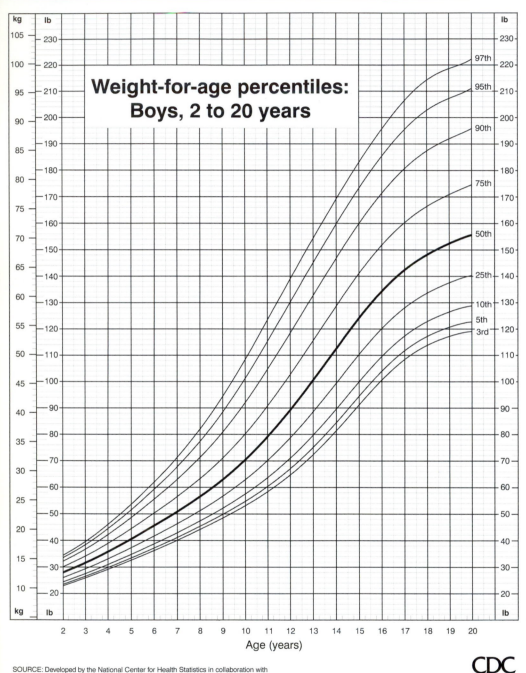

Weight-for-age percentiles: Boys, 2 to 20 years

SOURCE: Developed by the National Center for Health Statistics in collaboration with
the National Center for Chronic Disease Prevention and Health Promotion (2000).

CDC
CENTERS FOR DISEASE CONTROL
AND PREVENTION

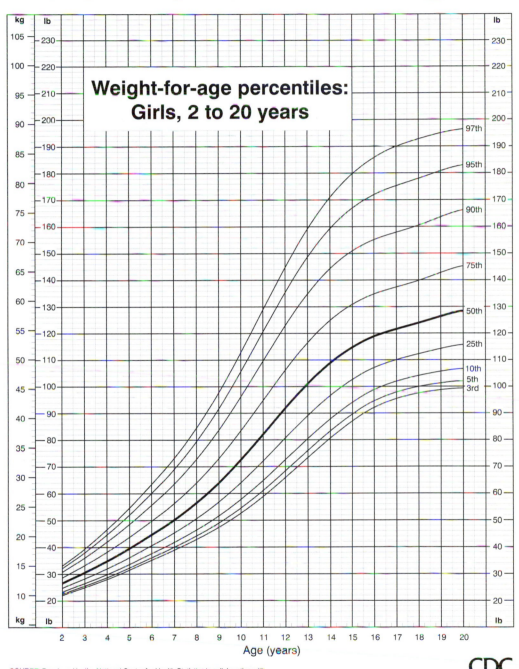

Weight-for-age percentiles: Girls, 2 to 20 years

97th
95th
90th
75th
50th
25th
10th
5th
3rd

Age (years)

SOURCE: Developed by the National Center for Health Statistics in collaboration with the National Center for Chronic Disease Prevention and Health Promotion (2000).

CDC
CENTERS FOR DISEASE CONTROL
AND PREVENTION

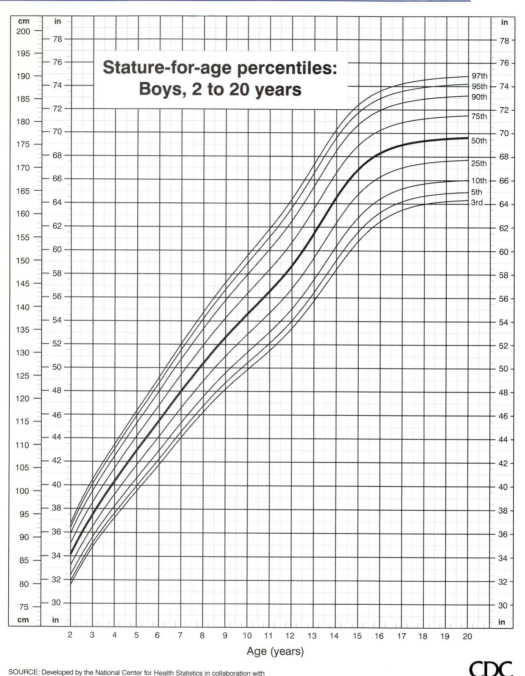

Stature-for-age percentiles: Boys, 2 to 20 years

SOURCE: Developed by the National Center for Health Statistics in collaboration with the National Center for Chronic Disease Prevention and Health Promotion (2000).

CDC
CENTERS FOR DISEASE CONTROL AND PREVENTION

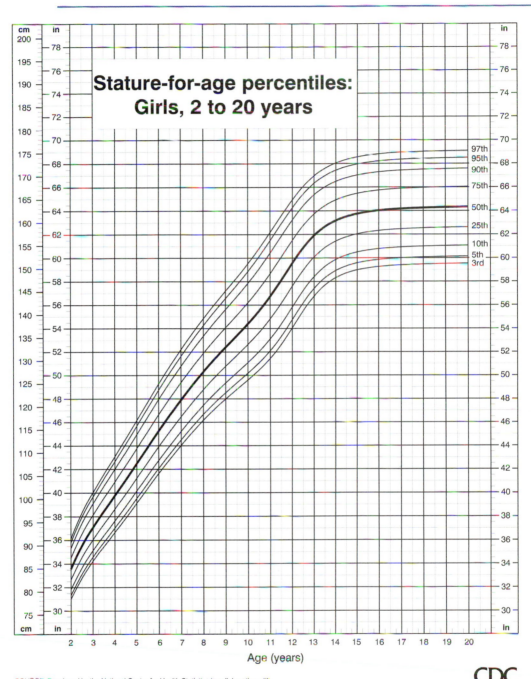

Stature-for-age percentiles: Girls, 2 to 20 years

SOURCE: Developed by the National Center for Health Statistics in collaboration with the National Center for Chronic Disease Prevention and Health Promotion (2000).

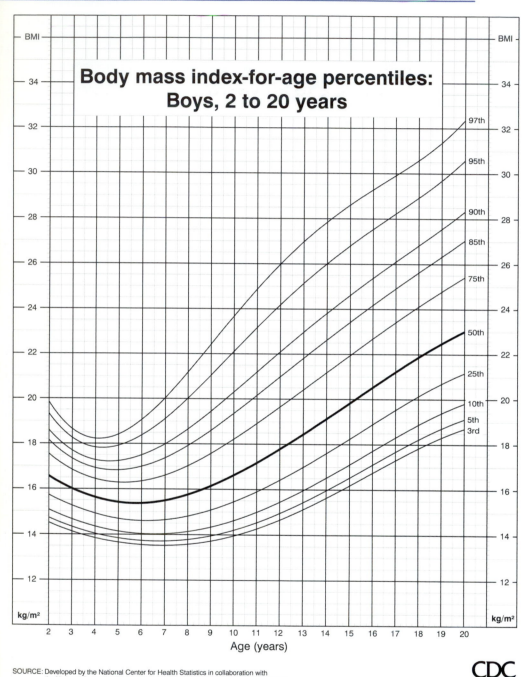

Body mass index-for-age percentiles:
Boys, 2 to 20 years

SOURCE: Developed by the National Center for Health Statistics in collaboration with
the National Center for Chronic Disease Prevention and Health Promotion (2000).

CDC
CENTERS FOR DISEASE CONTROL
AND PREVENTION

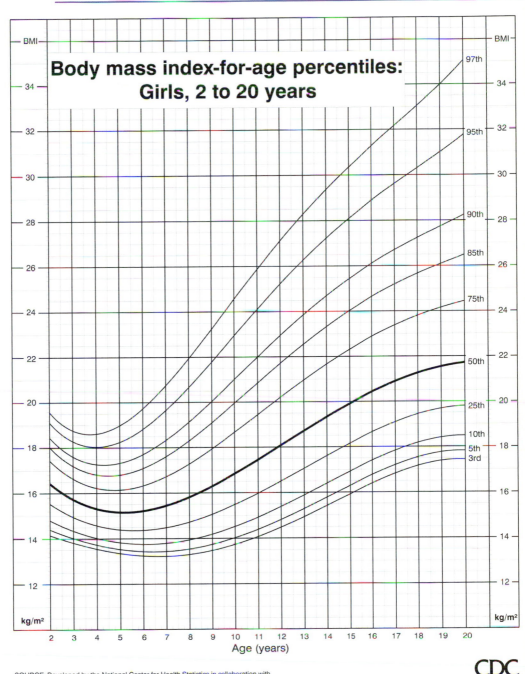

Body mass index-for-age percentiles:
Girls, 2 to 20 years

SOURCE: Developed by the National Center for Health Statistics in collaboration with
the National Center for Chronic Disease Prevention and Health Promotion (2000).

CDC
CENTERS FOR DISEASE CONTROL
AND PREVENTION

Glossary

Absorption The process of taking substances into the interior of the body.

Adaptive thermogenesis The change in energy expenditure induced by factors such as changes in ambient temperature and food intake.

Adenosine triphosphate (ATP) The high-energy molecule used by the body to perform energy-requiring activities.

Adequate Intakes (AIs) Intakes recommended by the DRIs that should be used as a goal when no RDA exists. These values are an approximation of the average nutrient intake that appears to sustain a desired indicator of health.

Adipocytes Fat-storing cells.

Adipose tissue Tissue found under the skin and around body organs that is composed of fat-storing cells.

Amino acids The building blocks of proteins. Each contains a carbon atom bound to a hydrogen atom, an amino group, an acid group, and a side chain.

Anorexia nervosa An eating disorder characterized by self-starvation, a distorted body image, and low body weight.

Antioxidant A substance that is able to neutralize reactive molecules and hence reduce the amount of oxidative damage that occurs.

Appetite The integrated response to the sight, smell, taste, or thought of food that initiates or delays eating.

Atherosclerosis A type of cardiovascular disease that involves the buildup of fatty material on the artery walls.

Basal energy expenditure (BEE) The minimum amount of energy that an awake, resting body needs to maintain itself. It is measured after 12 hours without food or exercise.

Basal metabolic rate (BMR) The rate at which energy is used by an awake, resting body to maintain itself.

Behavior modification A process used to change habitual behaviors gradually and permanently.

Bioelectric Impedance Analysis A technique for estimating body composition that measures body water by directing electric current through the body and calculating resistance to flow.

Body mass index (BMI) A measure of weight in relation to height that is used to compare body size with a standard.

Bomb calorimeter An instrument used to determine the energy content of food. It measures the heat energy released when a food is combusted.

Calorie The amount of heat needed to raise one gram of water 1°C (33.8°F). It is commonly used to refer to a kilocalorie, which is 1,000 calories.

Cholesterol A lipid made only by animal cells that consists of multiple chemical rings.

Daily Value A nutrient reference value used on food labels to help consumers see how foods fit into their overall diets.

Dietary Reference Intakes (DRIs) A set of reference values for the intake of nutrients and food components that can be used for planning and assessing the diets of healthy people in the United States and Canada.

Diet-induced thermogenesis The energy required for the digestion, absorption, metabolism, and storage of food. It is equal to approximately 10% of daily energy intake.

Digestion The process of breaking food into components small enough to be absorbed into the body.

Direct calorimetry A method of calculating energy use that measures the amount of heat produced by the body.

Doubly-labeled water method A technique for measuring energy expenditure based on the distribution of hydrogen and oxygen labeled with isotopes.

Electron transport chain The final stage of cellular respiration in which electrons are passed down a chain of molecules to oxygen to form water and produce ATP.

Elements Substances that cannot be broken down into products with different properties.

Glossary

Energy The capacity to do work.

Energy balance A state in which body weight remains stable because the amount of energy consumed in the diet equals the amount expended.

Enzymes Protein molecules that accelerate the rate of specific chemical reactions without being changed themselves.

Essential nutrients Nutrients that must be supplied in the diet because they cannot be made in sufficient quantities in the body to meet needs.

Estimated Average Requirements (EARs) Intakes recommended by the DRIs that meet the estimated nutrient needs (as defined by a specific indicator of adequacy) of 50% of individuals in a gender and life-stage group.

Estimated Energy Requirements (EERs) Energy intakes recommended by the DRIs to maintain body weight.

Fatty acid An organic molecule made up of a chain of carbons linked to hydrogens with an acid group at one end.

Fiber Nonstarch polysaccharides in plant foods that are not broken down by human digestive enzymes.

Free radical One type of highly reactive molecule that causes oxidative damage.

Gene A length of DNA that contains the instructions for making a protein.

Ghrelin A hormone produced by the stomach that helps regulate food intake.

Gluconeogenesis The synthesis of glucose from simple noncarbohydrate molecules. Amino acids from protein are the primary source of carbons for glucose synthesis.

Homeostasis A physiological state in which a stable internal body environment is maintained.

Hormones Chemical messengers that are produced in one location, released into the blood, and elicit responses at other locations in the body.

Hypothalamus The region of the brain that monitors and regulates conditions and activities in the body, including food intake and energy expenditure.

Indirect calorimetry A method of estimating energy use that compares the amount of oxygen consumed with carbon dioxide expired.

Insulin A hormone produced by the pancreas that is involved in blood sugar regulation.

***In vitro* fertilization** Process in which a woman's egg is fertilized by a man's sperm in a laboratory and is then implanted in the woman's uterus.

Isotope An alternative form of an element that has a different atomic mass, which may or may not be radioactive.

Ketone Molecule formed when there is not sufficient carbohydrate to completely metabolize the acetyl CoA produced from fat breakdown.

Ketosis A condition of excessive ketone levels in the blood.

Kilocalorie (kcalorie) The amount of heat required to raise the temperature of 1 kilogram of water 1°C (33.8°F).

Large-for-gestational-age A term for a baby born weighing more than 4 kg (8.8 lbs) at birth.

Lean body mass Body mass attributed to nonfat body components such as bone, muscle, and internal organs. It is also called fat-free mass.

Leptin A protein hormone produced by adipocytes that signals information about the amount of body fat.

Lipid A group of organic molecules, most of which do not dissolve in water. Lipids include fatty acids, glycerides, phospholipids, and sterols.

Macronutrients Nutrients needed by the body in large amounts. These include water and the energy-yielding nutrients—carbohydrates, lipids, and proteins.

Malnutrition Any condition resulting from an energy or nutrient intake either above or below that which is optimal.

Glossary

Menarche The onset of menstruation, which usually occurs between the ages of 10 and 15.

Metabolism The sum of all the chemical reactions that take place in a living organism.

Micronutrients Nutrients needed by the body in small amounts. These include vitamins and minerals.

Mucus A viscous fluid secreted by glands in the gastrointestinal tract and other parts of the body. It acts to lubricate, moisten, and protect cells from harsh environments.

Neurotransmitter A chemical substance that carries messages to and from the brain.

Nutrients Chemical substances in foods that provide energy, structure, and regulation for body processes.

Nutrition A science that studies the interactions that occur between living organisms and food.

Obese A condition characterized by excess body fat. It is defined as a body mass index of 30 kg/m^2 or greater or a body weight that is 20% or more above the desirable body weight standard.

Overnutrition Poor nutritional status resulting from a dietary intake in excess of that which is optimal for health.

Overweight A body mass index of 25 to 29.9 kg/m^2 or a body weight 10 to 19% above the desirable body weight standard.

Physical Activity (PA) value A numeric value based on typical activity level used in estimating energy expenditure.

Phytochemical A substance found in plant foods that is not an essential nutrient but may have health-promoting properties.

Protein-sparing modified fast A very-low-calorie diet of high protein content designed to maximize the loss of fat and minimize the loss of protein from the body.

Recommended Dietary Allowances (RDAs) Intakes recommended by the DRIs that are sufficient to meet the nutrient needs of almost all healthy people in a specific life-stage and gender group.

Resting energy expenditure (REE) An estimate of basal energy expenditure that has been measured after only a few hours without food or activity.

Resting metabolic rate (RMR) An estimate of basal metabolic rate that is determined by measuring energy utilization after 5 to 6 hours without food or exercise.

Satiety The feeling of fullness and satisfaction, caused by food consumption, that eliminates the desire to eat.

Saturated fat or **saturated fatty acid** A fatty acid in which the carbon atoms are bound to as many hydrogens as possible and that contains no carbon-carbon double bonds.

Starches Carbohydrates made of many glucose molecules linked in straight or branching chains. The bonds that hold the glucose molecules together can be broken by the human digestive enzymes.

Subcutaneous fat Body fat that is located just under the skin.

Sugars The simplest form of carbohydrate.

Thermic effect of food (TEF) or **diet-induced thermogenesis** The energy required for the digestion, absorption, metabolism, and storage of food. It is equal to approximately 10% of daily energy intake.

Tolerable Upper Intake Level (UL) The maximum daily intake by an individual that is unlikely to pose risks of adverse health effects to almost all individuals in the specified life-stage and gender group.

Total energy expenditure (TEE) The sum of all the energy needs of the body for a day.

Triglyceride (triacylglycerol) The major form of lipid in food and in the body. It consists of three fatty acids attached to a glycerol molecule.

Underweight A body mass index of less than 18.5 kg/m^2 or a body weight 10% or more below the desirable body weight standard.

Unsaturated fat or **unsaturated fatty acid** A fatty acid that contains one or more carbon-carbon double bonds.

Glossary

Very-low-calorie diet A weight-loss diet that provides fewer than 800 calories per day.

Visceral fat Fat that is located around internal organs.

Weight cycling The pattern of repeatedly losing and regaining weight.

References

Note: Once a reference has been cited, that same number is applied throughout the book to represent the same source.

1. Centers for Disease Control and Prevention. "Prevalence of Overweight and Obesity Among Adults: United States 1999–2000." Available online at *http://www.cdc.gov/nchs/releases/02news/obesityonrise.htm.*

2. Office of the Surgeon General. *The Surgeon General's Call to Action to Prevent and Decrease Overweight and Obesity.* Rockville, MD: U.S. Department of Health and Human Services, 2001. Available online at *http://www.surgeon-general.gov/topics/obesity.*

3. Hill, J. O., and J. C. Peters. "Environmental contributions to the obesity epidemic." *Science* 280 (1998): 1371–1374.

4. Young, L. R., and M. Nestle. "The contribution of expanding portion size to the obesity epidemic." *American Journal of Public Health* 92 (2002): 246–249.

5. Smith, G. P. "Control of food intake." *Modern Nutrition in Health and Disease,* 9th ed., eds. M. E. Shils, J. A. Olson, M. Shike, and A.C. Ross. Baltimore: Williams & Wilkins, 1999, pp. 631–644.

6. Rolls, B. J., E. L. Morris, and L. S. Roe. "Portion size of food affects energy intake in normal-weight and overweight men and women." *American Journal of Clinical Nutrition* 76 (2002): 1207–1213.

7. Hill, J. O., H. R. Wyatt, G. Reed, and J. C. Peters. "Obesity and the environment: Where do we go from here?" *Science* 299 (2003): 853–855.

8. Popkin, B. M., and C. M. Doark. "The obesity epidemic is a worldwide phenomenon." *Nutrition Reviews* 56 (1998): 106–114.

9. World Health Organization. "Controlling the Global Obesity Epidemic." Available online at *http://www.who.int/nut/obs.htm.*

10. Drewnowski, A., and B. M. Popkin. "The nutrition transition: New trends in the global diet." *Nutrition Reviews* 55 (1997): 31–43.

11. Vorster, H. H., L. T. Bourne, C. S. Venter, and W. Oosthuizen. "Contribution of nutrition to the health transition in developing countries: A framework for research and intervention." *Nutrition Reviews* 57 (1999): 341–349.

12. National Institutes of Health, National Heart, Lung, and Blood Institute. *The Practical Guide: Identification, evaluation, and treatment of overweight and obesity in adults.* NIH NHLBI, NIH Publication 02-4084, 2000.

13. Kuczmarski, R. J., et al. "Varying body mass index cut off points to describe overweight prevalence among U.S. adults: NHANES III (1988 to 1994)." *Obesity Research* 5 (1997): 542–548.

14. Snead, D. B., S. J. Birges, and W. M. Kohrt. "Age-related differences in body composition by hydrodensitometry and dual-energy x-ray absorptiometry." *Journal of Applied Physiology* 74 (1993): 770–775.

15. Fields, D. A., G. R. Hunter, and M. I. Goran. "Validation of the BOD POD with hydrostatic weighing: Influence of body clothing." *International Journal of Obesity and Related Metabolic Disorders* 24 (2000): 200–205.

16. Albu, J., D. Allison, C. N. Boozer, et al. "Obesity solutions: report of a meeting." *Nutrition Reviews* 55 (1997): 150–156.

References

17. Conway, J. M. "Ethnicity and energy stores." *American Journal of Clinical Nutrition* 62 (suppl) (1995): 1067S–1071S.

18. National Cancer Institute Cancer Facts. "Obesity and Cancer: Questions and Answers." Available online at *http://cis.nci.nih.gov/fact/3_70.htm.*

19. Key, T. J., N. E. Allen, E. A. Spencer, and R. C. Travis. "The effect of diet on risk of cancer." *Lancet* 360 (2002): 861–868.

20. Institute of Medicine, Food and Nutrition Board. "Dietary Reference Intakes for Energy, Carbohydrates, Fiber, Fat, Protein, and Amino Acids." Washington, D.C.: National Academies Press, 2002.

21. Schoeller, D. A. "Recent advances from application of doubly-labeled water to measurement of human energy expenditure." *Journal of Nutrition* 129 (1999): 1765–1768.

22. Friedman, J. M. "The alphabet of weight control." *Nature* 385 (1997): 119–120.

23. Schwartz, M. W., D. G. Baskin, K. J. Kaiyala, and S. C. Woods. "Model for the regulation of energy balance and adiposity by the central nervous system." *American Journal of Clinical Nutrition* 69 (1999): 584–596.

24. Woods, S. C., R. J. Seeley, D. Porte, and M. W. Schwartz. "Signals that regulate food intake and energy homeostasis." *Science* 280 (1998): 1378–1383.

25. Anderson, G. H. "Regulation of food intake." *Modern Nutrition in Health and Disease*, 8th ed., eds. M. E. Shils, J. A. Olson, and M. Shike. Philadelphia: Lea & Febiger, 1994, pp. 524–536.

26. Cummings, D. E., D. S. Weigle, R. S. Frayo, et al. "Plasma ghrelin levels after diet-induced weight loss or gastric bypass surgery." *New England Journal of Medicine* 346 (21) (2002): 1623–1630.

27. Batterham, R. L., M. A. Cowley, C. J. Small, et al. "Gut hormone PYY(3-36) physiologically inhibits food intake." *Nature* 418 (6898) (2002): 650–654.

28. Abernathy, R. P., and D. R. Black. "Healthy body weights: an alternative perspective." *American Journal of Clinical Nutrition* 63 (suppl) (1996): 448S–451S.

29. Tremblay, A., J-P. Després, G. Thriault, et al. "Overfeeding and energy expenditure in humans." *American Journal of Clinical Nutrition* 56 (1992): 857–862.

30. Gura, T. "Uncoupling proteins provide new clues to obesity's causes." *Science* 280 (1998): 1369–1370.

31. Levine, J. A., N. L. Eberhardt, and M. D. Jensen. "Role of nonexercise activity thermogenesis in resistance to fat gain in humans." *Science* 283 (1999): 212–214.

32. Robison, J. I., S. L. Hoerr, K. A. Petersmarck, and J. V. Anderson. "Redefining success in obesity intervention: The new paradigm." *Journal of the American Dietetic Association* 4 (1995): 422–423.

33. Stevens, J., J. Cai, E. R. Pamuk, et al. "The effect of age on the association between body mass index and mortality." *New England Journal of Medicine* 338 (1998): 1–7.

34. Wilmore, J. H. "Increasing physical activity: Alterations in body mass and composition." *American Journal of Clinical Nutrition* 63 (suppl) (1996): 456S–460S.

35. American Dietetic Association. "Position of the American Dietetic Association: Very-low-calorie weight-loss diets." *Journal of the American Dietetic Association* 90 (1990): 722–726.

36. Horten, T. S., H. Drougas, A. Brachey, et al. "Fat and carbohydrate overfeeding in humans: Different effects on energy storage." *American Journal of Clinical Nutrition* 62 (1995): 19–29.

37. Campfield, L. A., F. J. Smith, and P. Burn. "Strategies and potential molecular targets for obesity treatment." *Science* 280 (1998): 1383–1387.

38. Anderson, R. A. "Effects of chromium on body composition and weight." *Nutrition Reviews* 56 (1998): 266–270.

39. Kurtzweil, P. "Dieter's brews make tea time a dangerous affair." *FDA Consumer* 31: July–August, 1997. Available online at *http://www.fda.gov/fdac/features/1997/597_tea.html/*.

40. Flancbaum, L., and P. S. Choban. "Surgical implications of obesity." *Annual Review of Medicine* 49 (1998): 214–234.

41. National Center for Health Statistics. "Prevalence of Overweight Among Children and Adolescents: United States, 1999." Available online at *http://www.cdc.gov/nchs/releases/02news/obesityonrise.htm*.

42. U.S. Department of Health and Human Services, Centers for Disease Control and Prevention. National Center for Health Statistics CDC growth charts: United States, Advance Data, No. 314, June 8, 2000 (revised). Available online at *http://www.cdc.gov/growthcharts*.

43. Ernst, N., and E. Obarzanek. "Child health and nutrition: Obesity and high blood cholesterol." *Preventive Medicine* 23 (1994): 427–436.

44. Berenson, G. S., W. A. Wattigney, S. R Srinivasan, and B. Radhakrishnamurthy. "Rationale to study the early natural history of heart disease: The Bogalusa Heart Study." *American Journal of the Medical Sciences* 310 (suppl) (1995): 22S–28S.

45. Bao, W., S. A. Threefoot, S. R. Srinivasan, and G. S. Berenson. "Essential hypertension predicted by tracking of elevated blood pressure from childhood to adulthood: The Bogalusa Heart Study." *American Journal of Hypertension* 8 (1995): 657–661.

46. Must, A., and S. Anderson. "Effects of obesity on morbidity in children and adolescents." *Nutrition in Clinical Care* 6 (2003): 4–12.

47. Richardson, S. A., A. H. Hastorf, N. Goodman, and S. M. Dornsbusch. "Cultural uniformity in reaction to physical disabilities." *American Sociological Review* 202 (1961): 241–247.

48. Latner, J., and A. Stunkard. "Schoolchildren, stigma, and obesity." *Obesity Research* 9 (2001): 94S.

49. Hsu, L. K. "Epidemiology of the eating disorders." *Psychiatric Clinics of North America* 19 (1996): 681–7006.

50. Barlow, S. E., and W. H. Dietz. "Obesity evaluation and treatment: Expert Committee recommendations." The Maternal and Child Health Bureau, Health Resources and Services Administration and the Department of Health and Human Services. *Pediatrics* 102: E29, 1998.

References

51. Zive, M. M., H. L. Taras, S. L. Broyles, et al. "Vitamin and mineral intakes of Anglo-American and Mexican-American preschoolers." *Journal of the American Dietetic Association* 95 (1995): 329–335.

52. Kennedy, E., and J. Goldberg. "What are American children eating? Implications for public policy." *Nutrition Reviews* 53 (1995): 111–126.

53. Nutrition and Health Promotion Program, International Life Sciences Institute. "A survey of parents and children about physical activity patterns." September–October 1996.

54. National Association for Sports and Physical Activity. "Physical activity guidelines for preadolescent children." 1998.

55. Gortmaker, S. I., A. Must, and A. M. Sobol. "Television viewing as a cause for increasing obesity among children in the United States." *Archives of Pediatrics and Adolescent Medicine* 150 (1996): 356–360.

56. Sylvester, G. P., C. Achterberg, and J. Williams. "Children's television and nutrition: Friends or foes?" *Nutrition Today* 30 (1995): 6–15.

57. Andersen, R. E., C. J. Crespo, S. J. Bartlett, et al. "Relationship of physical activity and television watching with body weight and level of fatness among children: Results from the third National Health and Nutrition Examination Survey." *Journal of the American Medical Association* 279 (1998): 938–942.

58. American College of Sports Medicine. "Position stand: Weight loss in wrestlers." *Medicine and Science in Sports and Exercise* 28 (1996): ix–xii.

Abernathy, R. P., and D. R. Black. "Healthy body weights: An alternative perspective." *American Journal of Clinical Nutrition* 63 (suppl) (1996): 448S–451S.

Albu, J., D. Allison, C. N. Boozer, et al. "Obesity solutions: Report of a meeting." *Nutrition Reviews* 55 (1997): 150–156.

American College of Sports Medicine. "Position stand: Weight loss in wrestlers." *Medicine and Science in Sports and Exercise* 28 (1996): ix–xii.

American Dietetic Association. "Position of the American Dietetic Association: Very-low-calorie weight-loss diets." *Journal of the American Dietetic Association* 90 (1990): 722–726.

Andersen, R. E., C. J. Crespo, S. J. Bartlett, et al. "Relationship of physical activity and television watching with body weight and level of fatness among children: Results from the third National Health and Nutrition Examination Survey." *Journal of the American Medical Association* 279 (1998): 938–942.

Anderson, G. H. "Regulation of food intake." *Modern Nutrition in Health and Disease*, 8th ed., eds. M. E. Shils, J. A. Olson, and M. Shike. Philadelphia: Lea & Febiger, 1994, pp. 524–536.

Anderson, R. A. "Effects of chromium on body composition and weight." *Nutrition Reviews* 56 (1998): 266–270.

Bao, W., S. A. Threefoot, S. R. Srinivasan, and G. S. Berenson. "Essential hypertension predicted by tracking of elevated blood pressure from childhood to adulthood: The Bogalusa Heart Study." *American Journal of Hypertension* 8 (1995): 657–661.

Barlow, S. E., and W. H. Dietz. "Obesity evaluation and treatment: Expert Committee recommendations." The Maternal and Child Health Bureau, Health Resources and Services Administration and the Department of Health and Human Services. *Pediatrics* 102 (1998): E29.

Batterham, R. L., M. A. Cowley, C. J. Small, et al. "Gut hormone PYY (3-36) physiologically inhibits food intake." *Nature* 418 (6898) (2002): 650–654.

Berenson, G. S., W. A. Wattigney, S. R Srinivasan, and B. Radhakrishnamurthy. "Rationale to study the early natural history of heart disease: The Bogalusa Heart Study." *American Journal of the Medical Sciences* 310 (suppl) (1995): 22S–28S.

Bibliography

Campfield, L. A., F. J. Smith, and P. Burn. "Strategies and potential molecular targets for obesity treatment." *Science* 280 (1998): 1383–1387.

Centers for Disease Control and Prevention. "Prevalence of Overweight and Obesity Among Adults: United States 1999–2000." Available online at *http://www.cdc.gov/nchs/releases/02news/obesityonrise.htm.*

Conway, J. M. "Ethnicity and energy stores." *American Journal of Clinical Nutrition* 62 (suppl) (1995): 1067S–1071S.

Cummings, D. E., D. S. Weigle, R. S. Frayo, et al. "Plasma ghrelin levels after diet-induced weight loss or gastric bypass surgery." *New England Journal of Medicine* 346 (21) (2002): 1623–1630.

Drewnowski, A., and B. M. Popkin. "The nutrition transition: New trends in the global diet." *Nutrition Reviews* 55 (1997): 31–43.

Ernst, N., and E. Obarzanek. "Child health and nutrition: Obesity and high blood cholesterol." *Preventive Medicine* 23 (1994): 427–436.

Fields, D. A., G. R. Hunter, and M. I. Goran. "Validation of the BOD POD with hydrostatic weighing: Influence of body clothing." *International Journal of Obesity and Related Metabolic Disorders* 24 (2000): 200–205.

Flancbaum, L., and P. S. Choban. "Surgical implications of obesity." *Annual Review of Medicine* 49 (1998): 214–234.

Friedman, J. M. "The alphabet of weight control." *Nature* 385 (1997): 119–120.

Gortmaker, S. I., A. Must, and A. M. Sobol. "Television viewing as a cause for increasing obesity among children in the United States." *Archives of Pediatrics and Adolescent Medicine* 150 (1996): 356–360.

Gura, T. "Uncoupling proteins provide new clues to obesity's causes." *Science* 280 (1998): 1369–1370.

Hill, J. O., H. R. Wyatt, G. W. Reed, and J. C. Peters. "Obesity and the environment: Where do we go from here?" *Science* 299 (2003): 853–855.

Hill, J. O., and J. C. Peters. "Environmental contributions to the obesity epidemic." *Science* 280 (1998): 1371–1374.

Horten, T. S., H. Drougas, A. Brachey, et al. "Fat and carbohydrate overfeeding in humans: Different effects on energy storage." *American Journal of Clinical Nutrition* 62 (1995): 19–29.

Hsu, L. K. "Epidemiology of the eating disorders." *Psychiatric Clinics of North America* 19 (1996): 681–700.

Institute of Medicine, Food and Nutrition Board. "Dietary Reference Intakes for Energy, Carbohydrates, Fiber, Fat, Protein, and Amino Acids." Washington, D.C.: National Academies Press, 2002.

Kennedy, E., and J. Goldberg. "What are American children eating? Implications for public policy." *Nutrition Reviews* 53 (1995): 111–126.

Key, T. J., N. E. Allen, E. A. Spencer, and R. C. Travis. "The effect of diet on risk of cancer." *Lancet* 360 (2002): 861–868.

Kuczmarski, R. J., et al. "Varying body mass index cut off points to describe overweight prevalence among U.S. adults: NHANES III (1988 to 1994)." *Obesity Research* 5 (1997): 542–548.

Kurtzweil, P. "Dieter's brews make tea time a dangerous affair." *FDA Consumer* 31: July–August, 1997. Available online at *http://www.fda.gov/fdac/features/1997/597_tea.html.*

Latner, J., and A. Stunkard. "Schoolchildren, stigma, and obesity." *Obesity Research* 9 (2001): 94S1.

Levine, J. A., N. L. Eberhardt, and M. D. Jensen. "Role of nonexercise activity thermogenesis in resistance to fat gain in humans." *Science* 283 (1999): 212–214.

Must, A., and S. Anderson. "Effects of obesity on morbidity in children and adolescents." *Nutrition in Clinical Care* 6 (2003): 4–12.

National Association for Sports and Physical Activity. "Physical activity guidelines for preadolescent children." 1998.

National Cancer Institute Cancer Facts. "Obesity and Cancer: Questions and Answers." Available online at *http://cis.nci.nih.gov/fact/3_70.htm.*

National Center for Health Statistics. "Prevalence of Overweight Among Children and Adolescents: United States, 1999." Available online at *http://www.cdc.gov/nchs/releases/02news/obesityonrise.htm.*

National Institutes of Health, National Heart, Lung, and Blood Institute. *The Practical Guide: Identification, evaluation, and treatment of overweight and obesity in adults.* NIH NHLBI, NIH Publication 02-4084, 2000.

Bibliography

Nutrition and Health Promotion Program, International Life Sciences Institute. "A survey of parents and children about physical activity patterns." September–October 1996.

Office of the Surgeon General. *The Surgeon General's Call to Action to Prevent and Decrease Overweight and Obesity.* Rockville, MD: U.S. Department of Health and Human Services, 2001. Available online at *http://www.surgeongeneral.gov/topics/obesity.*

Popkin, B. M., and C. M. Doark. "The obesity epidemic is a worldwide phenomenon." *Nutrition Reviews* 56 (1998): 106–114.

Richardson, S. A., A. H. Hastorf, N. Goodman, and S. M. Dornsbusch. "Cultural uniformity in reaction to physical disabilities." *American Sociological Review* 202 (1961): 241–247.

Robison, J. I., S. L. Hoeer, K. A. Petersmarck, and J. V. Anderson. "Redefining success in obesity intervention: the new paradigm." *Journal of the American Dietetic Association* 4 (1995): 422–423.

Rolls, B. J., E. L. Morris, and L. S. Roe. "Portion size of food affects energy intake in normal-weight and overweight men and women." *American Journal of Clinical Nutrition* 76 (2002): 1207–1213.

Schoeller, D. A. "Recent advances from application of doubly-labeled water to measurement of human energy expenditure." *Journal of Nutrition* 129 (1999): 1765–1768.

Schwartz, M. W., D. G. Baskin, K. J. Kaiyala, and S. C. Woods. "Model for the regulation of energy balance and adiposity by the central nervous system." *American Journal of Clinical Nutrition* 69 (1999): 584–596.

Smith, G. P. "Control of food intake." *Modern Nutrition in Health and Disease,* 9th ed., eds. M. E. Shils, J. A. Olson, M. Shike, and A.C. Ross. Baltimore: Williams & Wilkins, 1999, pp. 631–644.

Snead, D. B., S. J. Birges, and W. M. Kohrt. "Age-related differences in body composition by hydrodensitometry and dual-energy X-ray absorptiometry." *Journal of Applied Physiology* 74 (1993): 770–775.

Stevens, J., J. Cai, E. R. Pamuk, et al. "The effect of age on the association between body mass index and mortality." *New England Journal of Medicine* 338 (1998): 1–7.

Sylvester, G. P., C. Achterberg, and J. Williams. "Children's television and nutrition: Friends or foes?" *Nutrition Today* 30 (1995): 6–15.

Tremblay, A., J-P. Després, G. Thriault, et al. "Overfeeding and energy expenditure in humans." *American Journal of Clinical Nutrition* 56 (1992): 857–862.

U.S. Department of Health and Human Services. Centers for Disease Control and Prevention, National Center for Health Statistics. CDC growth charts: United States, Advance Data, No. 314, June 8, 2000 (revised). Available online at *http://www.cdc.gov/growthcharts*.

Vorster, H. H., L. T. Bourne, C. S. Venter, and W. Oosthuizen. "Contribution of nutrition to the health transition in developing countries: A framework for research and intervention." *Nutrition Reviews* 57 (1999): 341–349.

Wilmore, J. H. "Increasing physical activity: alterations in body mass and composition." *American Journal of Clinical Nutrition* 63 (suppl) (1996): 456S–460S.

Woods, S. C., R. J. Seeley, D. Porte, and M. W. Schwartz. "Signals that regulate food intake and energy homeostasis." *Science* 280 (1998): 1378–1383.

World Health Organization. "Controlling the Global Obesity Epidemic." Available online at *http://www.who.int/nut/obs.htm*.

Young, L. R., and M. Nestle. "The contribution of expanding portion size to the obesity epidemic." *American Journal of Public Health* 92 (2002): 246–249.

Zive, M. M., H. L. Taras, S. L. Broyles, et al. "Vitamin and mineral intakes of Anglo-American and Mexican-American preschoolers." *Journal of the American Dietetic Association* 95 (1995): 329–335.

Further Reading

WEIGHT MANAGEMENT

American Psychiatric Association. *Diagnostic and Statistical Manual*, 4th ed. Washington, D.C.: American Psychiatric Association, 1994.

Andersen, R. E., C. J. Crespo, S. J. Bartlett, et al. "Relationship of physical activity and television watching with body weight and level of fatness among children: Results from the Third National Health and Nutrition Examination Survey." *Journal of the American Medical Association* 279 (1998): 938–942.

Centers for Disease Control and Prevention. "Obesity and Overweight: A Public Health Epidemic." Available online at *http://www.cdc.gov/nccdphp/dnpa/obesity/index.htm*.

National Institutes Diabetes Digestive Kidney Diseases, Weight Control Information Network. "Statistics Related to Overweight and Obesity." Available online at *http://www.niddk.nih.gov/health/nutrit/pubs/statobes.htm*.

National Institutes of Health, National Heart, Lung, and Blood Institute. "Clinical guidelines on the identification, evaluation, and treatment of overweight and obesity in adults. Executive summary, June 1998." Available online at *http://www.nhlbi.nih.gov/guidelines/obesity/ob_home.htm*.

National Research Council. *Diet and Health: Implications for Reducing Chronic Disease Risk*. Washington, D.C.: National Academies Press, 1989.

Office of the Surgeon General. *The Surgeon General's Call to Action to Prevent and Decrease Overweight and Obesity*. Rockville, MD: U.S. Department of Health and Human Services, 2001. Available online at *http://www.surgeongeneral.gov/topics/obesity*.

Walsh, B. T., and M. J. Devlin. "Eating disorders: Progress and problems." *Science* 280 (1998): 1387–1390.

EXERCISE BENEFITS AND RECOMMENDATIONS

Albright, A., M. Franz, G. Hornsby, et al. "American College of Sports Medicine position stand. Exercise and type 2 diabetes." *Medicine and Science in Sports and Exercise* 32 (2000): 1345–1360.

American Dietetic Association. "Timely statement of the American Dietetic Association: Nutrition guidance for child athletes in organized sports." *Journal of the American Dietetic Association* 96 (1996): 610–611.

Andersen, R. E., C. J. Crespo, S. J. Bartlett, et al. "Relationship of physical activity and television watching with body weight and level of fatness among children: Results from the Third National Health and Nutrition Examination Survey." *Journal of the American Medical Association* 279 (1998): 938–942.

Centers for Disease Control and Prevention, U.S. Department of Health and Human Services. "Physical Activity and Health: A Report of the Surgeon General." 1996.

Haennel, R. G., and F. Lemire. "Physical activity to prevent cardiovascular disease. How much is enough?" *Canadian Family Physician* 48 (2002): 65–71.

"Nutrition and athletic performance—Position of the American Dietetic Association, Dietitians of Canada, and the American College of Sports Medicine." *Journal of the American Dietetic Association* 100 (2000): 1543–1556.

Pollock, M. L., G. A. Gaesser, et al. "ACSM Position Stand on the recommended quantity and quality of exercise for developing and maintaining cardiorespiratory and muscular fitness and flexibility in adults." *Medicine and Science in Sports and Exercise* 30 (1998): 975–991.

GENERAL NUTRITION

American Dietetic Association. "Americans' Food and Nutrition Attitudes and Behaviors—Nutrition and You: Trends 2002." Available online at *http://www.eatright.org/Public/Media/PublicMedia_10333.cfm*.

Cleveland, L. E., A. J. Cook, J. W. Wilson, et al. "Pyramid Servings Data Results from the USDA's CSFII, ARS Food Surveys Research Group." Available online at *http://www.barc.usda.gov/bhnrc/foodsurvey/home/htm*.

Food and Drug Administration, Center for Food Safety and Applied Nutrition. "A Food Labeling Guide. Appendix C, Health Claims, August 12, 1997." Available online at *http://vm.cfsan.fda.gov*.

Food and Nutrition Board, Institute of Medicine. "Dietary Reference Intakes for Calcium, Phosphorus, Magnesium, Vitamin D, and Fluoride." Washington, D.C.: National Academies Press, 1997.

———. "Dietary Reference Intakes for Energy, Carbohydrates, Fiber, Fat, Protein, and Amino Acids." Washington, D.C.: National Academies Press, 2002.

Further Reading

————. "Dietary Reference Intakes for Thiamin, Riboflavin, Niacin, Vitamin B-6, Folate, Vitamin B-12, Pantothenic Acid, Biotin, and Choline." Washington, D.C.: National Academies Press, 1998.

————. "Dietary Reference Intakes for Vitamin A, Vitamin K, Arsenic, Boron, Chromium, Copper, Iodine, Iron, Manganese, Molybdenum, Nickel, Silicon, Vanadium, and Zinc." Washington, D.C.: National Academies Press, 2001.

————. "Dietary Reference Intakes for Vitamin C, Vitamin E, Selenium, and Carotenoids." Washington, D.C.: National Academies Press, 2000.

Shils, M. E., J. A. Olson, and M. Shike, eds. *Modern Nutrition in Health and Disease*, 8th ed. Philadelphia: Lea & Febiger, 1999.

U.S. Department of Agriculture. "The Food Guide Pyramid." Home and Garden Bulletin No. 252. Hyattsville, MD: Human Nutrition Information Service, 1992; slightly revised, 1996.

U.S. Department of Agriculture, U.S. Department of Health and Human Services. "Nutrition and Your Health: Dietary Guidelines for Americans," 5th ed., 2000. Item Number 147-G. Hyattsville, MD: U.S. Government Printing Office, 2000.

Sarubin, A. *The Health Professional's Guide to Popular Dietary Supplements.* Chicago: American Dietetic Association, 2000.

WEIGHT MANAGEMENT

Financial costs of obesity
http://www.rand.org/publications/RB/RB4549

**Guidelines on the identification, evaluation, and treatment
of overweight and obesity**
http://www.nhlbi.nih.gov/guidelines/obesity/ob_home.htm

Prevalence of Overweight and Obesity Among Adults
http://www.cdc.gov/nchs/releases/02news/obesityonrise.htm

Statistics related to body weight
http://www.cdc.gov/nchs/releases/02news/obesityonrise.htm

**The Surgeon General's Call to Action to Prevent and Decrease
Overweight and Obesity**
http://www.surgeongeneral.gov/topics/obesity

Weight Control Information Network
http://www.niddk.nih.gov/health/nutrit/pubs/statobes.htm

GENERAL NUTRITION

American Dietetic Association
http://www.eatright.org

Americans' Food and Nutrition Attitudes and Behaviors
http://www.eatright.org/Public/Media/PublicMedia_10333.cfm

**Dietary Guidelines for Americans,
Food and Nutrition Information Center**
http://www.nal.usda.gov/fnic/dga/index.html

Dietary Reference Intakes, National Academies Press
http://www.nap.edu

Dietary Supplements
http://www.nutrition.gov

**Food Labeling, Center for Food Safety and Applied Nutrition,
U.S. Food and Drug Administration**
http://www.cfsan.fda.gov

Food Guide Pyramid, Food and Nutrition Information Center
http://www.nal.usda.gov/fnic/Fpyr/pyramid.html

Websites

Healthy Eating Index, Center for Nutrition Policy and Promotion
http://www.usda.gov/cnpp

**Nutrient content of foods using the Nutrient database for
Standard Reference, U.S. National Agriculture Library**
http://www.nal.usda.gov

The Vegetarian Resource Group, Information on Vegetarian Diets
http://www.vrg.org

World Health Organization
http://www.who.int

NUTRITION, HEALTH, AND DISEASE

American Cancer Society
http://www.cancer.org

American Heart Association
http://www.americanheart.org

Fight Back! Partnership for Food Safety Information
http://www.fightbac.org

Food Safety
http://www.foodsafety.gov

Healthy People 2010
http://www.health.gov/healthypeople/

National Center for Health Statistics
http://www.cdc.gov/nchs/

National Cholesterol Education Program
http://www.nhlbi.nih.gov/chd/

NUTRITION AND EXERCISE

Canada's physical activity guide
http://www.hc-sc.gc.ca/hppb/paguide

Typical activity patterns
http://www.ilsi.org/nhppress.html#2

Index

Index

page:

5:	AP Graphics	50:	Courtesy USDA
7:	AP Graphics	53:	Courtesy USDA
9:	AP Graphics	57:	Courtesy USDA
18:	AP Graphics	61:	© Jim Perkins
20:	© Duomo/CORBIS	63:	© Lester V. Bergman/CORBIS
23a:	© Frank Siteman / Index Stock Imagery	80:	© Jim Perkins
23b:	© Jim Perkins	89:	© Jim Perkins
25:	© Jim Perkins	112:	© Jim Perkins
36:	© Ed Quinn / CORBIS	117:	Courtesy CDC
43:	Lambda Science Artwork	122:	Courtesy USDA

Frontis 1: Agricultural Research Service, Photo by Peggy Greb
Frontis 2: Agricultural Research Service, Photo by Scott Bauer